THE POWER OF STYLE

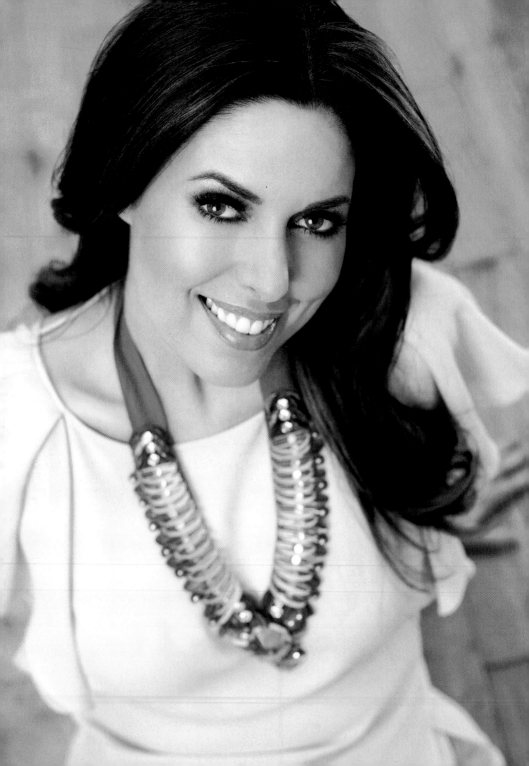

THE POWER OF STYLE

Everything You Need to Know Before You Get Dressed Tomorrow

Bobbie Thomas

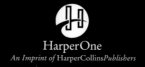

HarperOne

An Imprint of HarperCollins*Publishers*

HarperOne

Illustrations by Elizabeth Romaner

HarperCollins books may be purchased for educational, business, or sales promotional use. For information, please e-mail the Special Markets Department at SPsales@harper collins.com.

HarperCollins website: http://www.harpercollins.com
HarperCollins®, 📖 ®, and HarperOne™ are trademarks of HarperCollins Publishers.

FIRST EDITION

Designed by Kris Tobiassen

Library of Congress Cataloging-in-Publication Data

Thomas, Bobbie.
    The power of style : everything you need to know before you get dressed tomorrow / Bobbie Thomas. — First edition.
        pages cm
    ISBN 978-0-06-221974-9
    1. Women's clothing. 2. Fashion design. 3. Self-perception in women. I. Title.
    TT507.T4664 2013
    646.7'042—dc23   2012045933

13 14 15 16 17 RRD(C) 10 9 8 7 6 5 4 3 2 1

TO ANYONE ELSE WHO'S EVER FELT "LESS THAN" . . .
too short, too tall, too big, too small, too young,
too old, too weak, too bold, too odd, too plain, too shy,
or too vain—you are good enough, lovable,
and worthy of powerful style

CONTENTS

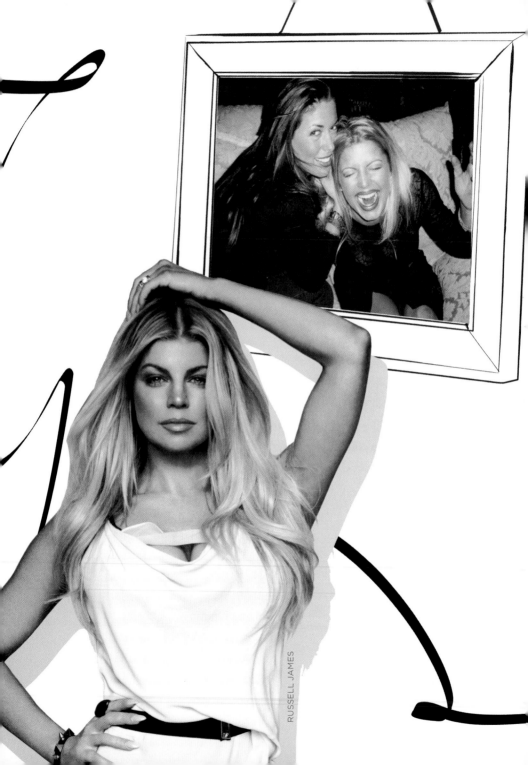

Foreword

BY FERGIE

Back in the late '90s, years before I joined the Black Eyed Peas, I was living in L.A. and working hard to help my all-girl group Wild Orchid break out into pop stardom. Just a few weeks after breaking up with my boyfriend of five years, my bestie, Eileen, introduced me to her sister Bobbie Thomas, who'd also just ended a five-year relationship. Even though our work lives couldn't be more different—Bobbie was counseling at a rape-crisis center; I was singing in a pop group—we ended up bonding over our breakups and helping each other work through the pain. Pretty soon we were spending most of our time together, sometimes just hanging out at each other's apartments or going out to dinner, and sometimes—that is, at least four nights a week—heading out to clubs like the Viper Room, Opium Den, Garden of Eden, Concord, the Lounge, Joseph's, Pop at AD, Firehouse, and Above Dublin's (to name just a few).

Bobbie turned out to be the best wingman a girl could ask for. We even had a secret code we'd use out in the clubs so that boys wouldn't know what we were talking about. One of my favorite things she told me about meeting men was to play it like a butterfly: instead of finding one guy you're into and hanging on to him all night, you should flutter around the room, land on one boy for a little while, then fly away again and see what else is out there. And if a guy was worth it, he'd end up chasing after you.

Back then Bobbie and I were both struggling to make a living doing what we loved. We didn't have a lot of extra cash to spend on clothes, so we had to get super creative when it came to style. We'd study fashion magazines and try to emulate the aspects of high fashion that really spoke to us, but always with our own quirky twist that had nothing to do with following trends. We were forever finding ways to reinvent and repurpose things to reflect whatever we were feeling at the time, like deconstructing a belt to turn it into a hair accessory, or cutting up tights and fishnets to wear as sheer sleeves.

But no matter what we had on when we headed out for the night, the key thing was to truly own what we wore—not just literally, but on a deeper, more powerful level that had everything to do with what made us unique as women. So while my look was more hip-hop and rocker and Bobbie's was about keeping it sexy in a sophisticated, upscale sort of way, in the end we complemented each other because we were both so true to our own personal style.

Self-expression was also at the heart of Bobbie's advice. One thing she always stressed to our girl gang was that staying true to yourself was the one and only way to find who (and what) is right for you. I learned from Bobbie that if you go out and take on some other persona to try to impress a guy, you're ultimately going to attract someone who isn't after the real you. By honoring your own uniqueness, you invite into your life not only the ideal man—but the best opportunities for you in general. You're also able to celebrate and embrace what's amazing about the women around you, rather than letting competition and jealousy get the best of you.

Empowerment was another message of Bobbie's that had a major impact on me then and still means so much to me today. Because of her experience as a rape-crisis counselor, she taught me everything about setting boundaries and watching out for myself and for my girl-friends. And even though we were all about going out and having fun night after night, Bobbie was also a very steadying influence for me—my therapist before I had an actual therapist. She'd studied psychology and had an incredible amount of knowledge about self-value and self-worth, and I soaked it all up like a sponge. I had self-help books and I had Bobbie, and I can't imagine having gotten through that time, and to where I am now, without her at my side.

The next best thing to having Bobbie as your own personal style guru, supporter, and partner-in-crime is having this book on your nightstand. *The Power of Style* builds on all that savvy and insight she passed on to me years ago in a way that's inspiring, empowering, and nothing short of life-changing.

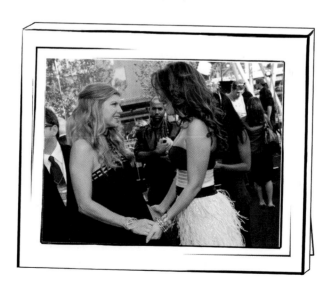

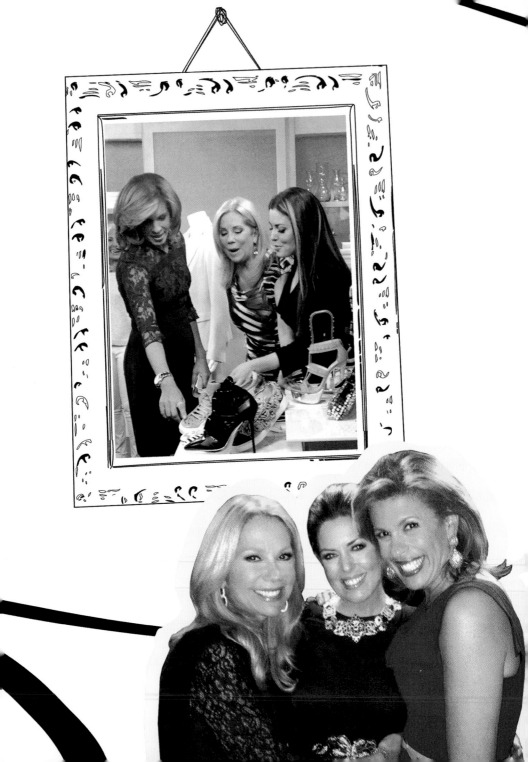

Foreword

BY KATHIE LEE GIFFORD AND HODA KOTB

You know the Bobbie T. you see on *TODAY*—sexy, stylish, and smart—but we know the Bobbie T. behind the scenes and she is so much more.

Bobbie has a true heart for helping women find the strength and courage they need to succeed in a stressful, complicated world. She believes she can help them and so do we, because we've watched her do it. What Bobbie seems to understand innately is the "psychology of style"—how your personal style affects you and how it affects all the people that you want to, in turn, affect.

Sound complicated? Not when you read what Bobbie has to say in her book. She makes it easy and understandable and she *doesn't judge you* if you don't happen to look like an über-model. What Bobbie helps you realize is that each woman is a "fierce force of nature in feminine form" with her own unique contribution to make in this world.

You're beautiful! You're valuable! You're one of a kind!

And, okay, you probably need a little help discovering all that.

So let her help you find your own special, sensational style.

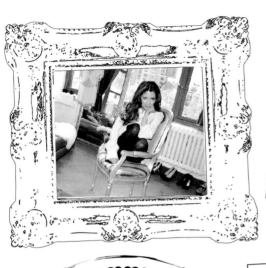

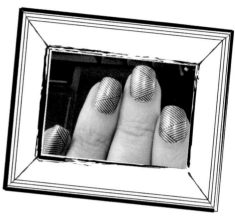

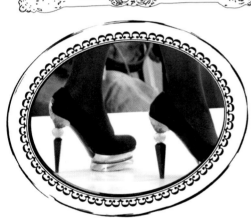

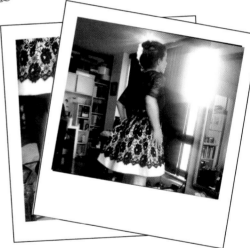

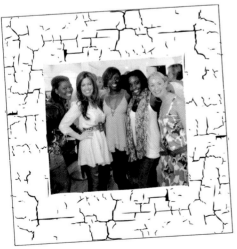

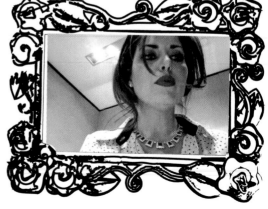

INTRODUCTION

Did you get dressed this morning? Yes, of course you did, because in our society you can't live your life naked. And even if you could, I think most of us would opt for clothing. After showering or brushing your teeth, dressing is probably the first thing you do every day. But have you ever stopped to consider that it's also the most important? This one act affects everything else that follows, yet the duty of putting something on is often left to the last few minutes before you have to run out the door.

> **Style is the way we speak to the world without words.**

Style is the way we speak to the world without words. Our style is a layer of language we wear and the first thing people notice about us. It's how we initially attract others, from potential mates to employers to friends. Family, coworkers, companions, and, most important, acquaintances and strangers are constantly "listening" to how we present ourselves, because our style is such an echo of who we are. I believe everyone has a "style speak" that is uniquely their own. Though we might not always realize it, we buy and wear clothes that physically represent and communicate our insights, frustrations, fears, goals, and desires. We then carry these signifiers into a workplace, a party, or on a date. Everyone gets dressed and most often with a purpose—whether they are conscious of it or not. We can miss out on some amazing opportunities if we forget or ignore the fact that appearances matter and if we overlook how others interpret them.

> I'm not here to tell you what your message should be, just that you need to have one.

I've met some truly amazing and accomplished women and men in my life, and the most noticeable trait they share is that they all have their own authentic sense of style. However, they didn't just stumble upon their statement by following someone else's opinions about what's stylish or by following trends. They understand exactly who they are and how to express that, each of them a unique, complete, and brilliant package in which the outside perfectly matches the inside. Much like products whose branding attracts the ideal consumer, we too can attract what we want through what we wear.

Are you covering up what you're trying to say to the world or perhaps advertising to the wrong audience? *The Power of Style* is about aligning your image—the one you see *and* the one others see—with your goals. Your style speak is a louder "voice" than anything you might scream from a rooftop, and the way you look says something to the world. So if you've succumbed to the mentality that your appearance doesn't matter, you've also agreed that your voice doesn't deserve to be heard. I'm not here to tell you what your message should be, just that you need to have one. And more specifically, it should be a message you've consciously developed and learned to express with style.

Though news and entertainment media usually interchange the terms "fashion" and "style," I believe these terms are not synonymous. Fashion alone is an external thing, not a way to identify you. Style, however, is about being whole and balanced. Whether I'm on NBC's *TODAY* show talking about the latest trends or hosting events at JCPenney or Gucci, I believe in leading a woman toward discovering her authentic self—her personality, her essence—on the inside and then reflecting that self on the outside through style. Unlike many fashion pundits out there, my "makeovers" are more about self-discovery and reinvention than over-hauls and major transformations. And when I offer fashion or beauty advice, it's mainly about adapting trends to fit a life-style that's genuine to the woman wear-

> **Style is about a lot more than stuff.**

ing them. The most stylish people I know are comfortable in their skin, and their clothes reinforce that. I love a hot shoe or a stunning gown as much as the next girl, but style is about a lot more than stuff.

In these pages I don't present overly simplified categories (classic, trendy, diva, glam, and so on), call out your lamest fashion mistakes, or offer an endless or regurgitated list of must-have pieces. Instead, I plan to get to know *you*. Seriously. You may think a book is inherently one-sided, but I have filled these pages with insightful questions and targeted exercises I call "style sessions," which I promise will make this process unique to you.

I divided *The Power of Style* into two equally important sections: part I's internal makeover and part II's external makeover, each comprised of five key steps. In part I, you'll learn to truly see yourself accurately (step 1), harness your body language to ensure effective first impressions (step 2), take control of your "style speak" (step 3), then understand your own worth (step 4) so you make a plan to fully commit (step 5). In part II, once you have a clearer understanding of who you are and what you want to say to the world, we'll get into how you can best say it with your style by identifying your best colors (step 6), selecting the most flattering clothes for your individual shape (step 7), editing your closet (step 8), interpreting your wardrobe needs (step 9), and, finally, learning how to shop smart (step 10). Because I couldn't ship myself to your house to physically go through this process with you, a book was the next best thing.

I've probably seen more women naked than most rock stars, both physically and emotionally. And this book is a result of stepping outside myself to capture my own thought process while styling them—the automatic mode I shift into in a dressing room, at a fitting, or in a friend's bedroom. While the "style therapy" I use may be instinctive for me at this point, I believe anyone can apply these methods to improve his or her image. By following the ten steps laid out in these pages, you will ultimately become a master at balancing your internal self-image with your external public image. It's all about drawing style *out* of you, instead of imposing it *onto* you. I believe progress and evolution can happen without assuming that the starting point is a bad one or that I'm the final word on taste. I plan to arm you with information about yourself, offer you a way to share it with the world, and show you how it can help attract your best life. And even if you think fashion is frivolous, overwhelming, scary, or—worst of all—unnecessary, I will prove that its value is often underestimated and empower you to express your most authentic self with every outfit every day.

As a style editor, an overwhelming majority of the questions I am asked revolve around the why and how of style. In this book, I will illuminate the *why* in part I and then explain the *how* in part II, so you'll first understand why you should care about your image and then learn how to make the right changes to improve it. Many of us are familiar with the mind–body connection, but when it comes to style, the focus is almost always disproportionally on the body. In order for part II to really work, it is essential to understand your emotional reasoning and motivation in part I. When doing makeover segments on television, I have advised producers many times to *not* start at the mall. Inevitably, the transformation will look good on camera, but it won't stick. The same can be said of anyone embarking on a lifestyle change who reaches for his or her wallet first. Buyer's remorse is a real thing, and any woman out there who has ever tried a fad diet (I'm not alone here, right?) knows that looking for a quick fix never works. You have to understand why you want to make changes and feel motivated to commit before positive, long-lasting effects can be seen. You don't start at the store; you start with yourself.

While I've always possessed a love for fashion, beauty, and the DIY approach, this is not where I got my start or even where I thought I would be today. My career began in the classroom, working on my graduate studies in marriage, family, and child counseling. When many of my friends in Los Angeles were forming pop bands, getting their acting careers off the ground, and networking with agency executives into the wee hours of the morning, I invested my time at a rape-crisis facility. For many people, including myself, the evolution from my work as a counselor to style guru on TV seemed like a drastic and perhaps even incongruent career transformation. And though the process wasn't deliberate or even conscious, I went along with it with little or no resistance because it somehow felt so organic, real, and natural.

My career trajectory was punctuated for me while on the set of an Alicia Keys photo shoot in New York City. A longtime photographer friend happened to be booked for the shoot; I was there to interview Alicia for the Style network. My friend and I hadn't seen each other for a few years, and after our hugs and kisses, he made a reference to knowing me as far back as when I was working at an HIV pharmacy and counseling at a rape center. Several people within earshot had almost audible thought bubbles and bewildered facial expressions that screamed, "Wow, she was helping HIV patients and rape survivors and now she's interviewing pop stars about their clothes?" However, as I stood in front of the camera with Alicia discussing style with her, it all came full circle for me. I asked her my questions, which admittedly are a little different from those of most television personalities: not just "What are you wearing?" but "Why are you wearing it? What does style mean to you? How has your style evolved? How do your talents connect to your self-expression?" Her responses were articulate, and she identified and shared how she uses her music, acting, clothes, and accessories to project a piece of her soul. In that moment I was reminded of how my particular style philosophy is truly about helping women discover this reality for themselves and live happier, more expressive lives. I'm still counseling. And while the subject matter may not be quite as heavy as it once was, it is equally significant. I'm still dealing with self-esteem, communication, attracting love, positive self-image, and contentment.

Over the past fifteen years, I've written advice columns, held style seminars, hosted shopping events across the country, and worked as a spokesperson for various powerful, female-centric campaigns. These experiences have afforded me the opportunity to connect with hundreds of thousands of women. As the style editor for NBC's *TODAY* show, I've had the unique good fortune to reach millions every week across every platform. While sharing my style philosophy with everyone from tweens to small-town homemakers to urban professionals to retired grandmothers, I've found that nearly every woman I meet identifies with my message as a fellow traveler on their own style journey and as a modern woman living in a modern woman's world. While the women themselves are always changing, my message has remained the same: style and psychology are intrinsically linked, and the better you feel about how you look and the message you are sending the world, the more confident, powerful, and ultimately happy you will be.

> **Style and psychology are intrinsically linked, and the better you feel about how you look and the message you are sending the world, the more confident, powerful, and ultimately happy you will be.**

My hope is that you will curl up on an overstuffed sofa with *The Power of Style* and never doubt that I'm right there with you—as a style guide, as a professional girlfriend, and as a cheerleader rooting for each one of you, *as* one of you. And when you finish this book, after having completed your inner and outer makeovers, I want your family, friends, boss, and strangers to immediately, and finally, see *you*—not a Gap ad or a celebrity wannabe or some designer's esoteric inspiration for that season. I want you to be your own muse, and I want to be the one who shows you how.

PART I

CHANGE STARTS WITHIN

Before I can help you with the pretty packaging, I need to know what's on the inside. Let's get to know you.

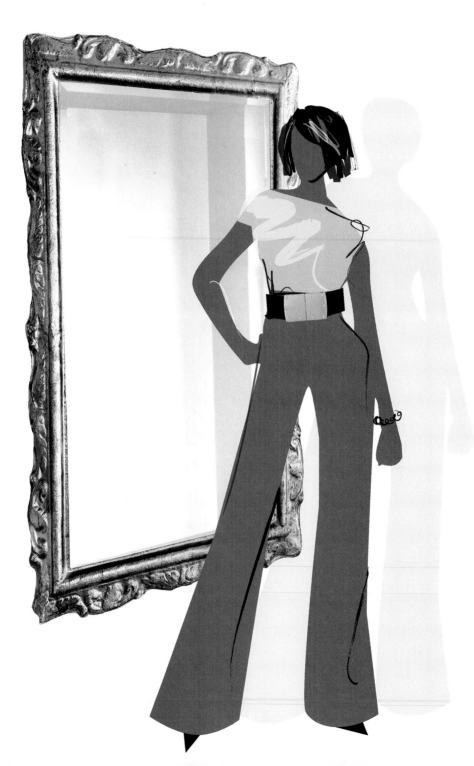

SEE YOURSELF

Take a Look in the Mirror

Have you ever wondered if you turn heads for the right reason? If you display an accurate impression of yourself when you enter a room? For a glimpse into the messages you send to the world, all you need to do is look in a mirror. And I mean that in the nicest way possible.

Most of us use mirrors—in our homes, in store dressing rooms, in our cars—to show us what we look like and ultimately determine how we feel about ourselves. Literally (and a little metaphorically), mirrors reveal and conceal, reflect and deflect, and exaggerate and diminish the image in front of us. Mirrors can make us laugh or cry, and under pressure, they can either crack or transform. As someone who dispenses style, fashion, and beauty advice for a living, I happen to work in an industry that's completely obsessed with mirrors—and sometimes for the wrong reasons. This experience has given me a lot of time to think about them. Whether you're drawn to mirrors or try to avoid them, mirrors can help us see ourselves more clearly.

Who's That Girl?

Find a mirror—preferably the one you spend the most time in front of—and get ready to get real. What do you see in the mirror? I want you to jot down the first five things that come to mind. It can be something you notice about your body or something you feel about yourself. For instance, is there a physical trait that stands out to you? Is there a knee-jerk emotion you feel when looking at yourself? Immediately write down whatever you notice, and be honest with yourself. It's really important to capture what you see and feel, as this will help you identify your perception.

1. _____

2. _____

3. _____

4. _____

5. _____

Though most of you are accustomed to thinking about mirrors of the framed, beveled, and gilded varieties, more figurative mirrors are all around you. The people, places, and events in your life act as mirrors too. Like a well-focused camera, a mirror captures an immediate and accurate glimpse of who you are at the time. Mirrors reflect images, and images reflect self-expression. And true self-expression is achieved through an authentic sense of style.

MIRROR, MIRROR ON THE WALL

When you look in a mirror, I know what you do. You focus on a pimple, crow's-feet, too-fair skin, or too-many freckles. You suck in your stomach. You push up your boobs and pull down your shirt. And then you sigh as if it's all a big, fat lost cause. Be honest. Did you just do any of these things when answering the style-session questions? Something similar?

Well, guess what? I know what you do because I do these things too. (By the way, so do supermodels and A-list celebrities.) Even after a facial, I head to a mirror to carefully examine every last pore. But just because we have similar habits doesn't mean they're healthy for our sense of self or sense of style. If there's anything I've learned from working with women, it's that we approach mirrors like we're on a search-and-destroy mission, as if mirrors exist only to show us what's wrong. We walk up looking for all those things we need to "fix" before we are suitable to leave the house, go into a meeting, or return to the dinner table. We seek out every imperfection, every flaw, and then—*kaboom!*—demolish our self-worth with thoughts about how we just don't measure up. I mean, have you ever met a woman who steps in front of a mirror with the intention of listing all the things she *likes* about herself? Who goes into the bathroom just so she can spend a few moments admiring herself? Our wonky motives remind me of the FX television show *Nip/Tuck,* where the handsome plastic surgeons famously begin each episode with the phrase "So tell me what you *don't* like about yourself?" That question struck such a chord with me, because it's something I've come to realize all women ask themselves every day—whether we know it or not. It's critical to identify and understand this reflex so we can change our behavioral instincts. Over one hundred years ago, long before the term "law of attraction" was popular, a man named Prentice Mulford wrote a book titled *Thoughts Are Things*. The basic gist was that we attract what we emanate. So the first step toward creating a positive outer image is to start manifesting a healthier inner one. Use this book to learn how to become your own secret admirer, by appreciating all your wonderful attributes (physical and otherwise). Others will follow your example.

You may have noticed that the title of this section is taken directly from *Snow White and the Seven Dwarfs:* "Mirror, mirror on the wall, who is the fairest one of all?" Every day, the evil queen anxiously awaited the answer, hoping it would be "you." But her magical mirror was a source of external validation. The truth is, we can be our own secret admirers by allowing the voice that responds to the fairy-tale question to be our own. Many of us feel it's too egotistical or self-centered to allow this voice to be heard. Au contraire, sister! This healthy, intrinsic self-esteem is the foundation we need. What you see is what others hear.

So what are you communicating to the outside world? Glance over the list you just made in the style session. Are these the positive message points you strive to promote and embody? If your answer is yes, then you already have a great foundation for us to build upon. If no, don't worry. *The Power of Style* will help get you there!

I've yet to meet a person, male or female, who looks in a mirror and likes what he or she sees 100 percent of the time. On those days when you just don't feel your best, your attitude shifts. As a resident of Manhattan, I'm surrounded by reflective surfaces all day long. On the street, there are store windows and glass buildings. I live in a modest-size apartment with mirrors galore—on my furniture and on my walls from floor to ceiling, which is an old design trick to help a room look bigger than it is. At work, I'm made up in front of mirrors, the TV monitors on set are mirrors, and I watch myself on video playback to critique my own segments, which is like watching myself through a mirror that adds ten pounds and often exaggerates flaws. Sounds fun, right? What makes any mirror especially precarious, though, is that the way we feel about ourselves when we're in front of it can seep into other areas of our lives when we step away. My everyday workspace happens to be directly across from a huge floor-to-ceiling mirror, and more times than I would probably like to admit I've been guilty of being a Debbie Downer, complaining aloud about my appearance. While, at the time, I don't realize my self-deprecating comments are affecting anyone other than myself, whoever I'm in the room with responds to my negative thoughts. Additionally, I'm often tempted to cancel an after-work event or an appearance if I feel like I'm not looking my best. I think this happens to many women all the time, and this sort of butterfly effect can potentially harm productivity or even result in missed opportunities.

> **What you see is what others hear.**

The bottom line is your self-esteem influences your spirit, and if you don't like yourself, everything about you will show it. The thing is, you'll never improve your life by focusing on your flaws. Picking at your face has never healed a breakout, and looking for cellulite doesn't exactly make you want to eat vegetables for dinner. You're more likely to plop down on the couch and feel sorry for yourself after one of those I-suck sessions and hope a cupcake or pint of ice cream will boost your spirits. On the other hand, when people feel great, that's when they're motivated to take better care of themselves.

That's when they have the confidence and self-awareness to make the changes they need to make.

The cool thing about mirrors is that because they produce an image in one moment, your reflection always has the chance to change and improve, and when it does, make way for an exhilarating high. Of all the makeovers I've worked on, my favorites are those where the subject isn't allowed to look in a mirror until it's over. This powerful moment is captured on air and the big reveal happens for the subject at the same time it does for the viewers. The woman absolutely glows when asked to step in front of a mirror for the first time, and the audience lights up too, because they feel and feed off her positive energy. There's an exciting synergy between the happiness she feels on the inside and the beauty they see on the outside. The reveal acts like one big mirror, bouncing and reflecting positive energy all around.

My friend Megan is a publicist, and she works tirelessly behind the scenes to protect and promote the images of her celebrity clients. She recently got engaged and asked me to be one of her bridesmaids. A few weeks after her announcement, I—along with a few of her other bridesmaids—accompanied her on a trip to the famous New York City bridal store Kleinfeld Bridal (yep, home of the TLC network's *Say Yes to the Dress*) to try on wedding dresses. We both have demanding careers and our work can consume our lives. This mentality was made even more evi-

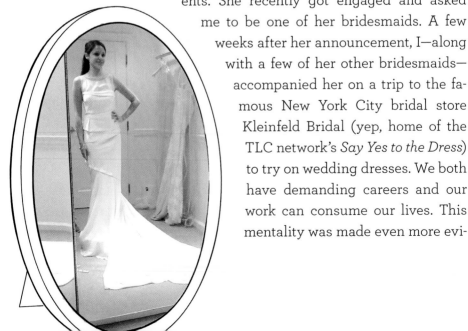

dent when Megan stepped out of the dressing room. We were all taken aback by how stunning she looked; the dress was breathtaking. But we could all tell she was uncomfortable being center stage. Even though this was her day to stand out, she was so used to building up other people that her immediate reaction to the attention was to hesitate. However, as soon as she stood in front of the mirror and saw herself put up on a pedestal, literally and figuratively, her whole attitude shifted. She saw herself in the spotlight and allowed herself to shine for a while. And we all loved seeing her beam. Her reaction was contagious and lifted all our spirits.

While both the televised makeover and wedding-dress shopping trip are unique examples of a special moment in someone's life, as you look in your own mirror every day, you can employ the same mindset and learn to love what you see.

By the time you finish this book, I promise you'll look in mirrors and not only see the positive but also celebrate your reflection every day. Right now some of you try to hush your inner voice from paying you compliments, because you think it's egotistical or self-centered to appreciate what you look like. Even worse, your negative self-talk may be so loud you can't even hear this voice in the first place. But that inner voice is a healthy self-esteem trying to break through and the foundation you need to be your most stylish, confident self.

THE OTHER MIRRORS AROUND US

As I mentioned earlier, not every mirror in your life is a glass one. The people, places, and events that are part of your everyday schedule are also effective mirrors. In fact, they can be far more revealing.

A Stickie a Day Keeps Buzzkills Away

I encourage you to stick a colored Post-it note to something personal you'll see first thing in the morning and possibly throughout the day (preferably your bathroom mirror; or if you share one and want this to be more private, it can be your wallet, phone, iPod, etc.). Song lyrics that have touched you, a simple reminder to smile or remember that you are loved, or even an inside joke that makes you giggle—all are little things that can make a big difference in your attitude on a daily basis. I happen to be a huge fan of famous sayings, like George Bernard Shaw's "Life isn't about finding yourself. Life is about creating yourself." Powerful quotes not only inspire you, but can also make you realize other people have felt the same way or faced the same challenges.

Notice how these small notes shift your mood and can both alter your experiences with others and trigger different outcomes.

Your partner, best friend, coworkers, even your hairdresser—the people with whom you choose to surround yourself have a lot to say about who you are and what you care about. In a perfect world, you'd only invite good people mirrors into your world. You know who I'm talking about: those rare and special gems who act like the magical mirrors in a boutique that make us look taller, thinner, and somehow just a little bit better. Often you're at your most beautiful through someone else's eyes, because they know you well enough that they see all of you—your true spirit. My mother is like this for me. Ever since I was a little girl, I could do no wrong in her eyes. She has always made me feel special and important. Even now, with us living on opposite coasts (I live in New York and she lives in LA), she takes time to e-mail me after nearly every television appearance to say I did a great job, even after those instances when I know I didn't. I could fall down on the red carpet or have a wardrobe malfunction on live TV and my mom would tell me no one had ever done it better. And while she has always made me feel beautiful as well, most of her encouragement and compliments have nothing to do with how I look.

Think of someone in your life who makes you feel this way. For example, how would you describe your best friend? If I were to describe mine, my immediate reaction would be to tell you he is a contrast in motion. The same day he was excited to show me the "baking room" in his house, he forgot to tell me he also bought a new shotgun. Honestly, he could be a whole other book, so let's get back to your BFF. Are the adjectives that come to mind describing personality traits or physical attributes? Our friends and loved ones remember our thoughtfulness, sense of humor, and acts of kindness long before they hold us accountable for gaining five pounds or wearing white pants after Labor Day.

Now, compare these to a bad mirror, one that warps or distorts your image. Sometimes you have people in your life who reflect negative images of yourself back to you. If you've ever had a boss who belittled you, a significant other who made you feel inferior, or a jealous friend, you know what I'm talking about. Even the most sacred of bonds, a mother–daughter relationship, may need perspective. A critical parent may have the best of intentions, but not realize the effect of his or her feedback.

It's heartbreaking to watch someone go from feeling invincible to insecure in a matter of moments. I've often been witness to how the "advice" or "two cents" a loved one offered can reflect back disappointment to a young girl or woman looking in this mirror. We are conditioned to trust comments from close friends and family, but it is important to be aware of angles that might bend or twist the reflection. People who make you feel negatively about yourself are like mirrors under unflattering lights, or set at the wrong kind of tilt, which makes you look shorter than you are. They can bring you down. They also reveal a lot about what you accept and expect from yourself and others. Plus, they can eventually harm your self-respect.

The best scenario is to surround yourself with people mirrors who, first, accurately reflect who you are and, second, see you the same way you see yourself, warts and all. Have you ever felt excited to meet a colleague's best friend and then been shocked when you finally do, because she's critical, negative, or bitchy? You might think, "Of all the people out there, *that's* who she chose as her bestie? Wow." While it's a commentary on the friend, it speaks even greater volumes about your colleague; in many ways it's an extension of your colleague's own overall style or self-expression.

If you have negative people mirrors in your life, how do you get rid of them? Well, acknowledging you don't have complete control over many of the individuals you encounter every day—including coworkers, in-laws, and even certain social acquaintances—there are still ways to diminish the effects their distorted reflections have on your sense of self. It's all about awareness. Imagine, again, that these folks are literal mirrors. They are the reflective surfaces you know to avoid: the mirrored windows in your office's lobby, which stretch you out, or a puddle of water in the street presenting your blurry image. You know these reflections aren't accurate—that's why you never get ready for an important event in your office lobby or haul your makeup bag outside when it rains. Distorted people mirrors should be viewed similarly. You might walk through that lobby every day and chances are you will continue to see your reflection in various pools of water now and again, but these are not the mirrors you trust. They should have little or no bearing on how you view yourself. Being aware of the people in your life who reflect who you really are, as well as those who don't, helps you choose to spend your time cultivating more positive relationships and reflections.

On another note, peer pressure is a common theme for teenagers but it can also be an issue for many adults. While we all strive to be individuals, we also feel the need to fit in. Are you trying to keep up with the Joneses? Is the designer bag or shoes you splurged on a status symbol for others to take note of, or is it a special investment that means something to you and puts a punctuation mark on your personality? While it's natural for friends to have common tastes, you run the risk of

> "It's good to be different. No one ever stood out in a flock."
>
> —Lynn Harless

getting lost in the crowd, not having your own voice, and not attracting what you may really want. It's important to be true to who you are and identify the difference between conforming and having the courage to be quirky. You don't want to be a mirror image of anyone else. To quote one of my best friends—and one of the wisest women I know—Lynn Harless, "It's good to be different. No one ever stood out in a flock."

ACTIONS SPEAK LOUDER THAN WORDS

Beyond people, your emotional reactions to situations and your life-style are also mirrors of who you are. They illustrate choices you've made, and your choices indicate what you hold dear. How you treat others, how you treat yourself, and even how you enter a room are all mirrors of self-expression. The way you respond to a challenging situation is a powerful mirror too—whether you're personable, kind, vulgar, calm, polite, or graceful.

In terms of lifestyle, I'll never forget the first time I bumped into a friend from college and she invited me to her apartment for coffee. She looked terrific, and her home was neat and well decorated. When we talked about her job and love life, she had it under control,

STYLE SESSION

Who Are Your People?

Make a list of the five people with whom you spend most of your time. These are very telling figurative mirrors in your life. Next to each name, use two adjectives to describe the person and then two words about how he or she makes you feel. For example, when I think of my friend Maggie, I think "loyal" and "smart"; the way she makes me feel is "happy" and "grateful." And when my father comes to mind, I think "concerned" but also at times "critical." As I was growing up, he made me feel "loved" but also "imperfect." As you now know, the ways in which other people make you feel can significantly affect your self-perception, either positively or negatively.

Take a look at your list. Are the adjectives you wrote down the words you would want people to describe you with? After all, these people surround you. Do they make you feel better about yourself or worse? If the answer to any of these top five is worse, consider whether you can limit the amount of time you spend with that person. If not, move forward through this book armed with the awareness that this particular person is an inaccurate reflection of who you are or who you want to be. We've all been hurt or wounded at one point or another in life. But remember, the more you pick a scab, the more permanent the scar becomes. You have complete power and control over whether or not you choose to pick at your scabs. The same is true about the people in your life you invest in.

Once you identify any people who may be warping your positive self-image, you can consciously begin to limit the amount of influence you allow them to have over your sense of self and, in turn, your style.

(A daughter's note: I love my father. He made me who I am today. I am very aware that parents most often do the best they can to help their children, and my dad has always supported me. However, even with the best of intentions, those closest to us can sometimes skew how we see ourselves. So it is important to be open and honest when doing this exercise.)

1. _____

2. _____

3. _____

4. _____

5. _____

and for the stuff she couldn't manage, she certainly had a healthy perspective. I felt energized just being around her. I had a total girl crush and couldn't wait to hang out again. When I recapped the afternoon to some mutual friends, they'd all had similar experiences with her. She was consistent and lovely, and everything about her—the way she looked, lived, spoke, acted—all mirrored who she was. She had an authentic flow, because her personality matched the exterior world she had created for herself. Plus, because she was so secure and content in that world, I felt really good in her company. There's comfort in transparency and authenticity. When you invest energy in your home, your relationships, and yourself, you celebrate your spirit in a way that tells others who you are in a genuine, contagious, and exciting way.

If I were to crash your next birthday bash, dinner party, or home-renovation project, what would the mirrors in your life say about you? Try to step outside yourself and examine your clothes, where you live, your relationships, your job, your body, your daily interactions, your finances—it's like looking into a giant mirror. The way others see you and the way you treat them are also reflections of who you are. So go on. Take a good look around you. It's tough to be objective about something so personal, but nobody's here to judge you, and we can all stand to improve a bit. So be honest. Do you like what you see?

HOW ALL THESE MIRRORS INFLUENCE YOUR STYLE

As you now know, one of the best ways to explore and hone your style is to look at the multidimensional mirrors in your life. As I've said, style is how we speak to the world without words. It's how you visually present your inner self. Because so much of your style comes from clear and accurate self-expression, it's also the ability to feel comfortable in your own skin. You must be able to see yourself as you are before developing a style plan you can build from.

So when I talk about style, I'm talking about an image that feels real to you *and* resonates as genuine to others. When there is incongruence, you may find you are not saying what you want, which can result in your not getting what you want from life. For example, if you are single and hoping to meet someone, why wait for an actual date to put your best self together (do your hair, make up your face, and put some thought into your outfit) when right now, and every day, there are hundreds of people waiting to meet you? (Fun fact, statistically speaking: your odds of meeting someone are much higher when you're out in the world rather than in your apartment.) So if the mirrors in your life are showing you a person who isn't who you think you are or who you want to be, there's a good chance you're projecting a style that isn't your own, or at least not your most desired.

> **The definition of style is self-expression.**

Though I work in the fashion industry, for me style does not equal the latest trends or flashiest brands. Style is so much more powerful and personal. The definition of style is self-expression, so fashion and beauty are simply two of the many tools that help you communicate, through a common visual language, what you're all about—what you see in your ideal mirror. Being stylish is not about having a certain body type or bank account; it's about embracing your individuality and radiating that spirit in your work, relationships, and everywhere else. My goal is to help you use the external to amplify your internal messages. When you walk into a business meeting or cocktail party, I want you to feel self-assured and comfortable about how you look, because your clothes accurately support and express who you are.

Lots of us project a style that isn't our own. And despite what some stores, magazines, and reality shows would have you believe, style isn't about hiring a fashion expert to pick out your clothes, or stuffing your closet with designer samples that make you feel good about choosing the "right" look. As far as I'm concerned, you already have style. It just needs a little guidance.

> **Being stylish is not about having a certain body type or bank account; it's about embracing your individuality and radiating that spirit in your work, relationships, and everywhere else.**

If your best self—and therefore your public image—isn't honest and consistent with your style, it misrepresents who you are. It can also be distracting, since others might be confused about the type of person you are based on how differently you look and act. For example, it amused me to watch the way others reacted upon learning a middle-aged man dressed in a trendy trucker cap, T-shirt, and ripped jeans (usually accompanied by a female half his age) was actually the person responsible for negotiating and overseeing multimillion-dollar deals for a certain celebrity. While I had the chance to get to know this man and see firsthand that he was one of the best managers in the business, many people weren't sure if he should be taken seriously when they first encountered him. Is it emotionally ideal that we judge books by their covers? Of course not, but it's reality. Your appearance invites people to gauge your creativity, finances, charisma, sexuality, and background. Notice how none of these is about being trendy or fashionable. People use what you wear to glimpse into your soul, and if your style mirrors a healthy one, judgments don't have to be negative. Instead, they'll feel self-affirming and gratifying.

When you think about style as a reflection of who you are, how you live, how you feel, and what you want out of life, I hope the idea of honing it feels much less intimidating and significantly more valuable than when you first picked up this book. Having said this, I don't expect you to wake up tomorrow and magically feel amazing every time you look in the mirror. Rome wasn't built in a day. Even I'm still working to practice what I preach.

Secret Self-Esteem Booster

One of my all-time favorite viral videos is *Jessica's Daily Affirmation.* This video shows a young girl, Jessica, standing on her bathroom counter and looking into a mirror. Consumed with youthful joy and excitement (she's approximately five years old in the YouTube video), Jessica cheerfully lists all the things in her life she loves. Her list starts with family and friends (her dad, mom, cousins, aunts, sisters, etc.) and continues to physical attributes (her hair, haircut, pajamas) and wraps up with her exclaiming that she "can do anything good!" How can you not smile watching this little girl? Don't we wish we could all feel this way when we look in the mirror? Well, with a little practice, you can take a note from Jessica and get back to this place. Style is about more than just the physical; it's about your whole life. It's so much more than the reflection staring back at you; it's the sum of all the mirrors around you.

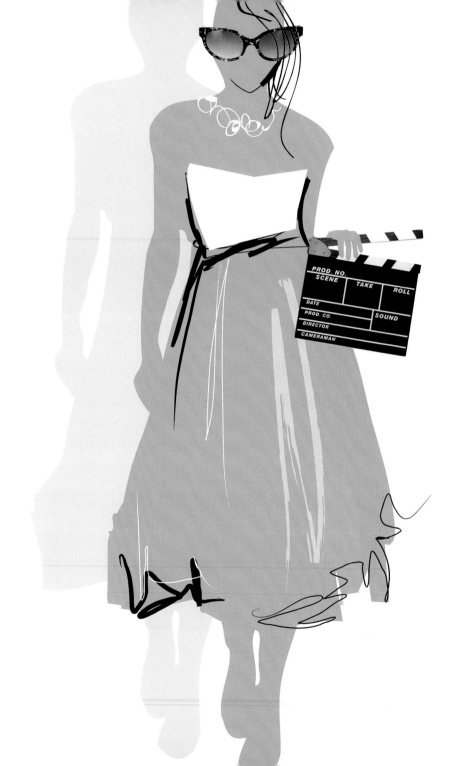

The clapperboard reads:

PROD. NO.

SCENE	TAKE	ROLL

DATE

PROD. CO.	SOUND

DIRECTOR

CAMERAMAN

ACT THE PART

Body Language and
First Impressions

Body language is a communication system that is collectively and individually more basic than the spoken or written word. That's why we intuitively understand that it's the most basic form of human communication.

—Peter A. Andersen, Ph.D.,
The Complete Idiot's Guide to Body Language

"A picture is worth a thousand words" and "It's written all over your face" are two phrases we've heard hundreds of times. They resonate with us because we understand what they are getting at—that you don't have to speak in order to get your point across. According to a study conducted by Dr. Albert Mehrabian at UCLA, 93 percent of communication is nonverbal. So what you're *not* saying is predominantly responsible for how you express yourself and ultimately how others view you. When you walk into a room, you deliver your message long before you ever say a word. Your style is literally a layer of language you wear. Yet we spend way too much time overanalyzing that remaining 7 percent. We're so caught up in what to say, what not to say, what he said or didn't say, we forget to pay attention to the primary, unspoken messages. I'll admit I've been guilty of being a 7-percenter. I've spent hours obsessing over words to use in almost every situation, from boring to death my best friend discussing every possible way I might say "hi" to a guy to carrying bullet points with me to confront a boss about a work conflict. How many lunches and phone calls with friends have you spent evaluating what he meant when he said such-and-such or what your boss's offhand comment meant? In reality, the actual words are often secondary. Imagine how this might apply to an important interview, a presentation, or a first date.

LET ME HEAR YOUR BODY TALK

So what are you really saying to the world, to your loved ones, and to yourself before you ever open your mouth? I learned a long time ago to "listen" to how people present themselves, because it's a much more accurate reflection of their true selves.

You notice other people's unspoken messages much more than you realize. Women are often referred to as communicators. When we are faced with a problem or have a decision to make, our first instinct is to talk about it with someone. Men might go into their caves to work things out internally, but women tend to find comfort in connecting to others. We are the talkative sex, and we use language

Flubbed First Date

A friend of mine recently went to a restaurant to meet a guy she had been set up with. She had heard great things about him from a mutual colleague and was assured they would have a lot in common and plenty to talk about. She took the time to plan a nice outfit in advance and got there early to find a good table. Her date, however, arrived late, wearing jeans and a wrinkled shirt, and proceeded to look at his cell phone frequently throughout the meal. She later recalled that they did, in fact, have many similar interests and the conversation was pleasant enough, but these nonverbal cues were what she ultimately used to decide that she wasn't interested in a second date.

as a method to build relationships, convey our wants and needs, and express ourselves. However, language is a very small part of how we communicate to the world around us; the nonverbal ways in which we express our style are equally, if not more, important. So why should we ever allow ourselves to be shamed for liking to shop, for caring enough to take two hours to get ready to go out, for painstakingly decorating our homes, or for any of the other countless self-expressions sprinkled throughout our lives? These actions are all forms of communication. I'm no scientist, but the way I see it, the female gender is biologically programmed to continually seek out just the right thing to wear or bring to any given occasion. Because these things—whether perfume or a present—ultimately help us convey even the smallest facet of our personalities and allow us to "say" something to others. (Taking all this into account, it makes me wonder, ladies: Is shopping our birthright?)

So, if you haven't already, allow yourself to embrace fashion and beauty as valuable parts of your life and self-expression. Think about how a friend's short, striking haircut, nail art, and bright wardrobe are all elements that help you understand more about her. The same goes for you, so you should take time to understand and invest in the things that help showcase your personality.

But it's not only the fashion or beauty aspects that communicate to the outside world. Think about when you are asked to describe someone. Do you immediately think "she always wears blue jeans" or "she loves the color pink"? While you may mention some of these physical preferences, more often than not you will start by saying she's "assertive" or "generous" or "camera shy." Self-expression is style. So, in ad-

New York: Old Stereotypes

Growing up in Los Angeles, I had many preconceived notions about the "typical" New Yorker. When I moved to New York in my late twenties, I expected most of the people I met in my new city would be assertive, fast talking, and dressed in black. Sure, this person definitely exists, but the friends I've made in New York over the past few years are almost nothing like this stereotype. I had assigned these traits and concocted these images in my head based on all the nonverbal representations I had seen in other people I knew from New York, coupled with the many portrayals we see in the media. The power of the unspoken had influenced my impressions before I even unpacked my first suitcase.

dition to your outside layer—your hair, makeup, and all the finishing touches—many aspects of your body language are also immediately apparent to others, who use them to make snap judgments about the kind of person you are. Your demeanor, posture, eye contact, facial expressions, how often you smile, or whether you fidget are all factored into your overall nonverbal message.

I've also come to realize that something as simple as social cadence goes a long way in influencing a personal impression. This revelation may seem like Manners 101, but it really speaks to someone's style. I have spent a lot of time in the South, and when I think of a typical Southern belle, I immediately envision a slower, easygoing sweetness and delicate mannerisms. Whenever I meet a woman from the South, I immediately transfer these traits to her, whether they are accurate or not. The nonverbal associations I have are strong. They are usually the first things we notice about someone and often the majority of what we take away after every encounter. This is why it's so important to be sure that the unspoken messages we are sending out are accurate expressions of who we are.

STAY IN SYNC

Understanding your body language is so important, because if your verbal and nonverbal channels of communication are out of sync, most people will rely on your nonverbal message and disregard what you're actually saying. Imagine that I came to your office, school, or PTA meeting to speak about this book. Obviously this topic is very special and important to me. I've devoted years to understanding the psychology of style and built a career around helping women understand how to use fashion and beauty as tools of self-expression. So if I arrived in sweatpants with messy hair and no makeup on and seemed distracted or tired while I was talking, do you think you'd believe what I was saying? Would you be excited to read this book? Odds are, probably not. My body language and overall appearance would conflict with my message. In circumstances like this, body language conveys much more than words can.

This sort of incongruence can clearly produce unintended results. Has there ever been a moment in your life when you were sure things were going to go one way and then the opposite occurred? Perhaps you had a job interview and felt you dazzled the boss with your articulate answers and impressive critical thinking, but then you never got a call for a second interview. Or maybe you had an amazing first date, but never heard from the person again. You could have gone over the experience in your head hundreds of times, and yet it still didn't make sense. In situations like these, it's highly possible you overlooked the power of the nonverbal. What you said during the interview or on the date may have been a perfectly accurate representation of who you are, your interests, strengths, and abilities. But if your body language was conflicting with these messages, game over!

While these are examples of your body language working against you and mixing your message to create potentially negative outcomes, the opposite can be true as well. These opportunities are what we're here to focus on. Now that you understand how powerful nonverbal communication is, you can start to use it to your advantage and ensure that you're always reinforcing your message. Think about the people in your life who have it all together (like my girlfriend from college in step 1). What they say, how they carry themselves, their body language, and their overall appearance are likely all aligned and consistent. Cohesive verbal and nonverbal messages communicate honesty, authenticity, and likability, because what they are saying is strengthened by *how* they are saying it. These are the people you want to be around and who others gravitate toward.

Something my friends often tease me about is that whenever I'm in an elevator, I always make eye contact with whomever I'm riding with and say hello. Depending on where you live, this may either seem completely normal or totally absurd. In Manhattan, we come into contact with so many people throughout the course of a day that I think people often forget this common courtesy. Maybe I'll get a very quiet "hi" from someone while they pretend to check their phone until the elevator door opens, but so much can be gained from genuinely connecting with people. More often than not, my simple action of looking at someone and saying "hello" or "how are you?" has had positive results. I'm confident it has everything to do with how my body language is reinforcing my greeting. If you smile, look that person in the eye, and say hello, the natural human reaction is to return the gesture.

The most attractive curve on your body is your smile. And this little act has led me to meet friends from all walks of life. For instance, all the models I use in my *TODAY* segments are women I've met organically via real-life circumstances. I ask friends, neighbors, and even women I meet on the street to showcase my looks, because I feel passionately that

> **The most attractive curve on your body is your smile.**

real women are the ones who actually wear the items I talk about. I have found many of my models by simply walking up to strangers, introducing myself, and inquiring.

Considering not everyone is immediately open to appearing live on national television, I have found that a friendly, genuine, warm demeanor goes a long way toward helping these women feel comfortable and open to the idea. By allowing my body language to reinforce my genuine intentions, the women are put at ease. Communicating, however, is a two-way street. I am far more likely to approach a woman who is projecting a positive vibe than one who is scowling and walking quickly past me with her head down.

Body language clearly affects us all. It's the only form of communication that is inevitable; no matter how hard we may try to conceal

Friendly Faces

Author Julie Muszynski, the famously beautiful gray-haired woman you can often see modeling for me in various capacities, was walking her dog through the hallway of my apartment building one day, and I was so taken with her look that I struck up a conversation with her. She had an effortless confidence about her and was immediately responsive and engaging. Her outward appearance and the way she carried herself were the first things I noticed about her, but after we began talking, I could tell that these initial impressions were reinforced by her inviting personality. This first meeting resulted in not only a professional relationship, but also a personal one. Now I consider Julie a good friend. When your body is in sync with what you're saying, you open yourself up to new possibilities and are much more likely to get your point across and get what you want from life.

Silence the Sound

Try watching your favorite television show on mute for five to ten minutes and observe the actors' body language. Take note of how each character either negates or reinforces what you know about their personalities and their goals during that episode. Actors are trained to use their entire bodies, along with their dialogue, to convince people of who they are and what messages they are trying to convey. So they are great examples of effective body language.

how we're feeling or what we're thinking, someone is interpreting a message from us at all times based on our mannerisms and overall demeanor. We can't turn these things off. But we can control what it is we're saying and learn how to leave a positive first impression that is representative of our individuality.

MAKE AN IMPRESSIVE FIRST IMPRESSION

Part of the reason we rely so much on body language and resort to "judging a book by its cover" is because that's all we have to go on in the beginning. Initially, someone is just "the girl in the red dress" or "the tall guy with the curly hair." But as we get to know people, we begin to identify them by their personality attributes, not their external qualities. It's these deeper reflections that are the truest. Have you ever had one of your best friends give you a gift accompanied by "This was just so *you*"? Well, what is it about that item that links it to who *you* are? What is your friend's perception of you that correlates to the color, use, design, or concept of that product? This is an example of how nonverbal messages emanate and communicate to the outside world, in almost every facet of our lives, who we are.

Why not use the external to amplify these core messages? What opportunities are we potentially missing out on because someone has a mistaken first impression of who we really are? When you know someone well—say a friend at work you see every day or your sister—most of the time you probably couldn't tell me what she's wearing, even if you just saw her. It's when you *don't* know someone that you notice everything about his or her appearance. So the way you look on the outside, along with your body language, is initially all you have to work with to ensure you are making a good first impression. What strangers see when they first meet you, and vice versa, is responsible for whether or not these people end up turning into friends. After all, the old cliché is true: you don't get a second chance to make a first impression.

So start paying attention. How do people react when you first make eye contact? What are the physical and verbal responses you elicit when you walk into a room? Are people responding to you or your designer handbag? How's your posture? Do you keep your eyes forward or do you tend to look at the ground when you walk? Do you exude confidence?

Ask yourself these questions (and if you're really feeling motivated and want to explore this deeper, ask a few close friends as well):

- **Are you confident and secure?** Do you own your space when you enter a social setting, or do you gravitate to a corner space or sink to the back to avoid attention?

- **Are you independent?** Do you move about on your own and feel comfortable walking to the bar, food buffet, or venture to find the restroom without a wing-woman?

- **Are you fun?** Whether you are required to be somewhere or not, do you find aspects to enjoy and make the most of a situation?

- **Are you a good listener?** Do you really hear what others say? Do you contribute enough, but not too much? Do you ask questions?

- **Are you fearful?** Do you engage with others or initiate conversation?

These are great questions to get you thinking about the kind of first impressions you may be making. How do you think your friends might answer these questions about you? These initial impressions stick, and unfortunately we human beings are pretty set in our ways once we form an opinion about someone. Furthermore, we tend to think that a behavior is an example of a person's permanent disposition. So the way you act upon first meeting is considered the way you always are. I think I can speak for everyone when I say that this is a terrifying thought. I have bad days when I'm not feeling like myself, and I shudder to think that I could be meeting people for the first time and giving them my worst for a first impression. Alas, these things occasionally happen. Fortunately, learning how to match your inner self to your outer self is the first big step toward minimizing these occurrences.

SEEING IS BELIEVING

Have you ever noticed the abundance of celebrity-endorsed advertisements? Everyone from Kim Kardashian to Betty White to Jay-Z to John Stamos has appeared in a commercial. Well, there's a simple reason for this and it's called the halo effect. As Dr. Peter A. Andersen describes it in his book *The Complete Idiot's Guide to Body Language*, it's when you form a positive impression of someone based on unrelated characteristics. We recognize these people, we like them, so we believe we'll like whatever they're selling. These famous faces are trustworthy experts to us, even though we don't know anything about who they really are as individuals. Our first impressions, based on the outward alone, have been formed and the reaction is good. The same can be said anytime we assume an attractive person is nice, an older person wise, or a redhead fun and sassy. The halo effect affects us all, and while it can extend beyond a person's physical appearance, it shows just how deeply what we see influences a first impression.

The flip side of this coin is when someone forms a negative assessment of you based on your outer appearance. Sadly, this happens all the time. As we've previously discussed, body language is an extremely powerful form of communicating, as is what you put *on* your body—your clothes, makeup, accessories, etc. If your appearance is misleading, it clouds or confuses the impression you make.

Take makeup, for example. Makeup is one of the greatest ways to express yourself. It is relatively inexpensive, easily accessible, and the fastest way to temporarily change your appearance. I love experimenting with beauty products, but I have learned firsthand

What's Your First Impression?

It's hard to ever really know what first impression you make. So why not turn to the power of the Internet to discover what physical impression you make on strangers? Hop online and visit bobbie .com/firstimpressions. Follow the instructions on the page to upload three photos of yourself (choose photos that depict you as you usually are—i.e., no professional photos, wedding pictures, or the like). Other visitors will then answer insightful questions below your photos to give you an idea of what impressions you make based on your image alone. This will give you an honest idea of how strangers perceive you and help you determine if you are accurately communicating on the outside who you are on the inside. Don't forget to share the love and write your impressions of others on the page!

how it can alter someone's perception of you. Whenever I am scheduled to appear on television, I spend an hour or so beforehand just doing my makeup (oh, how I miss the days before HDTV!). Walking around a TV studio, my made-up face looks completely normal, even at only six in the morning. Once I get home, I immediately change into comfier clothes and go about my normal day, but often without touching my face. Trust me when I say I have received some very odd looks from folks who see me at the grocery store at noon looking like I'm about to audition for a Broadway production. Suffice it to say, the messages makeup can send out into the world are powerful. And while makeup can conceal the things you want it to—a blemish or a dark spot, for instance—it can also conceal who you are and what you're trying to say.

How you dress works much the same way. Your clothing choices can make you appear confident, powerful, or desirable, or they can cause you to come off as unorganized, careless, or insecure. The quintessential example of this occurs during a job interview. (While many of you reading this may be either years into a career at one company or not working at all, this can apply to any circumstance

According to a 2011 study funded by Procter and Gamble and carried out by scientists at Massachusetts General Hospital, Harvard Medical School, Boston University, and the Dana-Farber Cancer Institute, researchers found that women who wear at least some makeup are viewed as more attractive, competent, and trustworthy than those without any makeup. However, using a varied scale, ranging from "no makeup" to "natural" to "professional" to "glamorous," the study also found that the subjects' positive perceptions of the women declined as the amount of makeup increased. While they still found these made-up women to be likable and attractive, they were thought to be less trustworthy. This study is just one example of how something as simple as makeup can appear to others as a shield, something you're trying to either hide behind or use to change who you are. It can help you appear strong and confident or insecure based on any number of factors, including where you are, who you are with, and whether it's day or night.

Care Doesn't Equal Cost

If you have a limited budget, I would much rather see you invest in a haircut and a new pair of shoes than a flashy suit. You wear your hair every day and, in addition to the extra confidence most women feel when they are sporting a new 'do, a good-looking coif shows that you pay attention to details. When it comes to shoes, many people overlook footwear in favor of what's up top. However, worn or scuffed shoes can come across as messy. You want your outfit to support what you're trying to convey rather than compete with it.

from which you are in a position to gain something.) When you're looking for a new job, your goal is to impress a potential employer. This person has never met you before, and the first impression you make is of the utmost importance. You'll want to make sure you wear something contemporary. This look comes across as informed, up-to-date, and speaks to what you offer as a candidate. If you appear dated, you may come across as behind the times, which can hurt your chances of being hired. This idea has nothing to do with being trendy, as a classic item like a blazer, a button-down blouse, or even a makeup choice can elevate your look. This is about taking time to think about what your clothing choice is saying. You want to demonstrate that you understand what's appropriate, taking into account the company's culture and making sure your image aligns with its brand.

EVERYDAY IMPRESSIONS

Aside from interviews, we all have numerous opportunities every day to make a first impression. We constantly have the potential to meet new people. Whether socially (at a party, reunion, baby shower, wedding) or professionally (while applying for a loan, meeting a co-op board, giving a presentation), the opportunity to make a good first impression probably arises far more often than you think. Two of the easiest and most effective questions I ask myself whenever I'm getting dressed for a specific occasion are:

1. Am I comfortable?
2. What word or sentence am I trying to convey?

The first question—Am I comfortable?—is one of the most important to consider before leaving the house. No matter where you're going, if you're physically uncomfortable in what you're wearing, it will show to other people. If your heels are too high, if your dress is too tight, even if you're wearing a lot of heavy accessories, it will reflect in how you walk, possibly cause you to fidget more than usual, or distract from what you're saying. The bottom line is that being uncomfortable will take away from your message.

Second, ask yourself what word or sentence you're trying to convey. This habit will go a long way in helping you decide if what you're wearing is appropriate and effective. If you have an appointment at a bank to discuss lowering your mortgage rates, you may want to channel the phrase "financially responsible." If, when you look in the mirror, you see nothing but jewelry and designer labels, rethink your outfit choice. To go on a hiking trip with friends, you may think "adventurous." You'll want your outfit to convey mobility and be colorful and unrestrictive. For a date, you'll likely want to appear warm and approachable.

These two questions are helpful when considering what your appearance says about who you are and what your ultimate goal is.

BRIDGING YOUR BODY AND MIND

The importance of body language cannot be overstated. It's the only constant, unavoidable form of communication, and you can—and should—use it to your advantage to strengthen your messages and help you achieve your goals. These nonverbal messages are inextricably tied to first impressions, and our first impressions often end up influencing whether we get that second interview, make a new friend, or meet our soul mates. We are judged, or at the very least interpreted, by the outside world based on how we look, whether we like it or not. We all want the fairy-tale ending, but we often forget that Cinderella didn't show up at the ball and sweep the prince off his feet wearing her work clothes and hiding in the corner wishing she were somewhere else. With a little help from her fairy godmother, she made a great first (physical) impression. It's not all about clothing, though. The mean stepsisters had fabulous gowns too, but it was Cinderella the prince fell for. This proves that we can't rely solely on looking great; we also have to *be* great. However, we sometimes miss out on opportunities when we ignore the simple truth that appearances matter . . . at least in terms of getting a foot in the door (or at the ball). It's important to know that style has both physical *and* emotional components. Learn to be aware of these messages and start noticing how others interpret them. This is what I call "style speak."

Sixty-Second Snapshots

For this style session, ask a favor of five friendly acquaintances, such as your local dry cleaner, friendly mail carrier, or grocery clerk. I like to call these individuals the sixty-second people in our lives, since we only see them a minute at a time. Using the survey below, write down your name or a phrase describing how this person knows you (e.g., "short brunette with the golden retriever who buys coffee from me every Saturday"). Then, ask them to take a minute and write down the type of impression you leave on them. To keep things easy, consistent, and anonymous, include a self-addressed stamped envelope with each survey. The feedback you receive is a helpful way to illustrate the kind of surface-level, nonverbal language you convey.

Snapshot Survey

How do you know me?

_____

_____

What do you think this person does for a living?

_____

_____

How old do you think this person is? _____

Is this person married or in a relationship? _____

Does this person have children? _____

On a scale of 1 to 6 (1=Strongly Disagree, 2=Disagree, 3=Neither Disagree nor Agree, 4=Agree, 5=Strongly Agree, 6=Not Applicable), rank the following traits regarding this person:

Confident _____   **Trustworthy** _____

Friendly _____   **Intimidating** _____

Intelligent _____   **Interesting** _____

Outgoing _____   **Shy** _____

Kind _____   **Generous** _____

Good sense of humor _____   **Good sense of style** _____

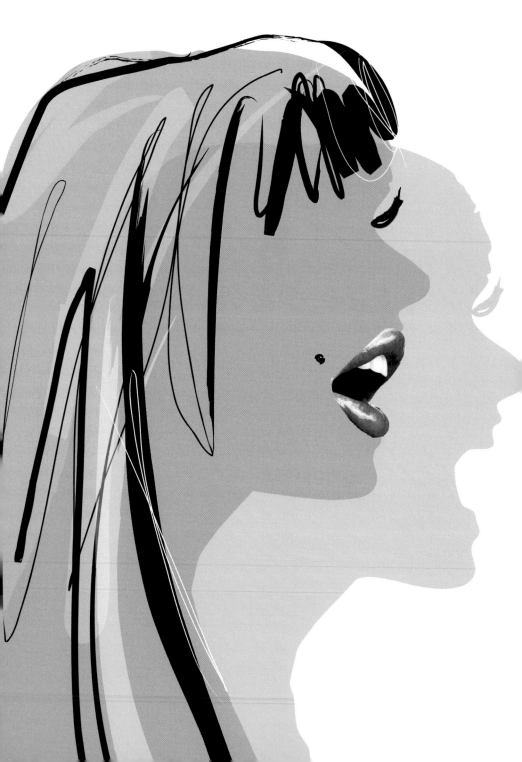

SPEAK UP

Brand Yourself

Now that we've established that style is self-expression and that it is communicated primarily to the outside world using nonverbal cues, such as body language and demeanor, it's time to assess what it is you're communicating with your fashion choices. What your style is saying is something I like to call your style speak.

As I've said, style is a layer of language you wear. Unlike verbal languages, however, style speak is universal. No matter where you are, your style is connecting you with others and giving insight into your personality, regardless of whether or not you actually speak the native tongue.

Understanding that the language you're wearing is constantly speaking on your behalf is only part of the process. Communication is a two-way street. In addition to the messages you put out, the way the world perceives those messages is equally important. And because your style speak is constantly being evaluated by the world, it's even more important to take advantage of what you can control.

From this step forward (in this book and in life), I want you to consider yourself a brand. Author and branding expert Marty Neumeier defines a brand as "a person's gut feeling about a product, service, or company." Therefore, *a personal brand is your distinctive perceived identity and intention. In other words, people's knee-jerk association to the experience of you*—the way you look, how you act, and whatever else they instantly recall when they see you or hear your name. What do the following names bring to mind: Marilyn Monroe, Oprah Winfrey, Lady Gaga, and you (insert your name here)? Quick, answer! This response is your current brand.

You are as worthy as any icon, celebrity, or Fortune 500 company to sell yourself. Style speak is how you put your brand out into the universe. So let's build your brand and advertise it accurately.

BUILD YOUR BRAND

Life is moving faster than ever, and thanks to technology (smartphones, instant uploading, live tweeting, text mania, and more), we as a society tend to look for shortcuts to quickly assess things and judge their worth, importance, and relevance in our lives. We can't help it. The purpose of branding is to make this process easier. For example, if I'm in a foreign country and in need of a cup of coffee, as soon as I see that familiar green Starbucks logo, I breathe a sigh of relief. I trust that logo, that brand, and I know what I'm getting when I see it. We make these associations with one another as well, and when you use style speak to clearly communicate a personal brand, you increase the chances of having others see you the way you want to be seen.

Iconic brands become familiar to us as their core identities are clearly and consistently conveyed. Take the ad campaigns of fashion designer Michael Kors, for example. These ads always get right to the heart of who the MK woman is. Regardless of the product being sold, whether fashion, accessories, or fragrance, the ads depict a glamorous, jet-setting lifestyle. A powerful, chic, on-the-go woman, usually stepping out of a private plane or luxury car, is bathed in a warm, golden glow and exudes an aspirational vibe. Guess ads are known for their signature black-and-white images, which play up a retro element complete with Bridget Bardot–style makeup and sexy, fun beach scenes. Bebe's dressed-up version of sexy pushes body-conscious clothing. The company has somehow figured out how to consistently sell a singular office-meets-the-club angle; when you see its ads you don't even need a logo to know "that looks like Bebe." Others like Tommy Hilfiger and Ralph Lauren, which may seem directed toward similar audiences on the surface, actually send out targeted, specific messages through their own unique versions of style speak. While both are anchored in Americana, Tommy Hilfiger's preppy visuals often include group shots of young people involved in collegiate outdoor activities. They evoke a type of Ivy League university feel, whereas Ralph Lauren focuses more on the individual, showcasing a sophisticated, country-club lifestyle.

The purpose of evaluating these ads is to get you thinking about the details, the layering in the messages, and how it all comes together to answer the question "Who is this brand?" The visual styling elements help tell the brand's story and get people to recognize it, ideally gaining the trust and favor of consumers. Similarly, using

"Who Am I?"

What story is your brand telling the world? Every day you make the decision to get out of bed, get dressed, and step outside. So, fortunately, every day you have the opportunity to strengthen your brand. Imagine for a moment that the paparazzi followed you around for a week, and then your pictures were published in a weekly magazine. Do you think the public would get an accurate idea of who you are? If your answer is yes, then your style speak is loud and clear. If your answer is no or you aren't sure, there are plenty of ways to speak up. Let's consider what your image is saying to others by asking two key questions: "Who am I?" and "What do I want to say?"

"Who am I?" can be an intimidating question. The answer comes down to your beliefs, values, likes, and dislikes. These answers are going to differ greatly for every reader, and that's one of the reasons I didn't begin this book with a list of ten items every woman must own. While these lists can be useful tools, they are often generic. It's important to approach them subjectively, so you can add your own spin or edit them to fit your lifestyle. As ancient philosopher Epictetus said, "Know, first, who you are, and then adorn yourself accordingly."

a holistic approach to creating your own cohesive personal brand can increase your self-confidence and your connection with others, heightening your presence and ultimately leading to personal and professional success.

In this section, I want to help you understand who you are by pointing out what you already know. Another reason it's so crucial to accurately know thyself is because, for good or bad, you will be stereotyped, numbered, assigned to mental boxes, and more. I'd like for you to mentally, verbally, and visually articulate exactly who you are, so you can take control of your own labels and influence the judgments passed.

> **"Know, first, who you are, and then adorn yourself accordingly."**
>
> **—Epictetus (AD 55–135)**

Let's go back to big brands for a moment. Think about the labels you gravitate toward, even if when just window-shopping. Pushing aside what's available to you, or what you can afford, what instinctively attracts you? Do you have one favorite or a few go-to retailers? If you have a particular designer or brand you wear more than most, it's likely because you resonate with that story. The portrayed aesthetic, values, and lifestyle align with yours, or at least with those you want to be associated with. If you consider yourself an equal-opportunity shopper and frequently visit a variety of retailers, think about what sections you are immediately drawn to. Even if you don't enjoy shopping, take note of any ads you like, what other women are wearing, including celebrities. All these hints can uncover more about who you are. Don't be discouraged if you find that what you are most attracted to isn't represented by your current style. The whole purpose of asking yourself these questions is to find out more about who you are, so you can build upon what you already have and continue to move from this point in the right direction. In part II, your answers to these questions will assist you in creating a wardrobe that will excite you and that you'll be proud of.

Create a Style File

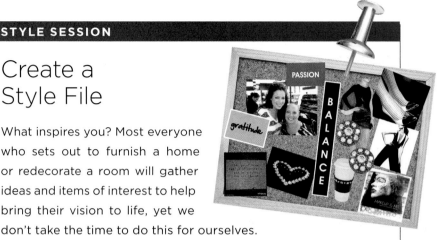

What inspires you? Most everyone who sets out to furnish a home or redecorate a room will gather ideas and items of interest to help bring their vision to life, yet we don't take the time to do this for ourselves.

Designers, editors, and stylists gather inspiration often in the form of a vision board. So for this style session, create your own style file. Collect pictures of your favorite people (yourself, friends, or celebrities), places, or things (furniture, food) that speak to you, as well as thought-provoking quotes and sentimental scraps. Tear out eye-catching ads or pages in magazines or catalogues. Be open-minded about where you draw from but selective in what you choose. This file will be a visual wellspring you can draw inspiration from to help you establish your brand, and you'll use style speak to reinforce it. I'm a big fan of the website Pinterest.com— an online pinboard where you can gather together all the things you love and share them with others. I have spent many hours browsing other people's boards, inspired by images or ideas they have pinned (see my page: Pinterest.com/BobbiesBuzz). Whether you decide to start a board on a site like Pinterest, keep your items in a physical file, save your items in an e-file on your computer, or paste them into a scrapbook or diary, make sure to choose whatever method is easiest and most accessible for you.

LOOK AND LISTEN

Your favorite movies can also reveal important elements of your personality. While writing this step, I shared this notion with my close friend Maggie, who initially scoffed at the idea, saying she didn't think her favorite movies had anything to do with her style. However, we kept talking and after just a few minutes she realized that not only is she drawn to a specific type of film (predominately movies about music or musicians) but also she has been taking fashion cues from them for years. She still covets Kate Hudson's coat from *Almost Famous*. I, on the other hand, have a wide range of favorite films that are representative of my eclectic sensibility. Baz Luhrmann's *Moulin Rouge* is a whimsical, fantastical film that speaks to my inner show-girl. Yet Woody Allen's classic *Annie Hall* is grounded very much in reality, set against the backdrop of the 1970s. While Diane Keaton's menswear-inspired wardrobe from the film has since become iconic, the plot also drew me in when I first saw it. The fast-talking, quick-witted dialogue and the New York City setting appealed to me, even as a teenager. Do you have any movies that resonate with you like this? When you identify with a story line or certain characters, and then see those things brought to life visually, the results can be transformative. Just ask any fan of *Sex and the City*. Fashion was often considered the fifth character in that show, and the wardrobe ultimately defined the female characters more than the dialogue.

The same can be said about books and music. When you read or hear something appealing, it conjures mental images and most of us instinctively think about how this content can be brought to life. I'm not the only one who has loved a song and mentally choreographed a corresponding music video in my mind, am I? The things you like reveal volumes about who you are and can help you more carefully craft your style speak. Try it yourself and write down a few of your favorite films, books, or songs in the space provided in the box below. These words will likely give you further insight into your own style speak.

Uncovering who you are can be a process, but chances are you already have a snapshot to work from. With over 700 million people using Facebook in 2012, I'm going to go out on a limb and say that a great many of you reading this book have created a Facebook profile at one point or another. If not, perhaps you've created a profile for a work directory, a dating site, or something similar. These

> **What is your favorite movie, book, and song? What adjectives do they make you think of that inform your style?**
>
> **Favorite Film:**
>
> **Adjectives:**
>
>
> **Favorite Book:**
>
> **Adjectives:**
>
>
> **Favorite Song:**
>
> **Adjectives:**

A Few of My Favorite Things

Everyone has been asked at one point or another "What items in your home would you grab if you had to make a hasty exit?" Most of us instinctively rattle off the obvious: family (of course), pets, pictures, laptop, and cell phone. Here, I would like you to answer this same question but without listing any of the above. (Don't worry. They are all safe.) This exercise will get you thinking about those superficial items that hold importance. Perhaps it's a piece of art, or your favorite scarf, sweater, or pair of shoes. Maybe it's something you've kept in your closet even though it no longer fits. Whatever these items are, think about why you would take them with you. Your answers may surprise you.

_____

_____

_____

_____

profiles include pictures, details about your life, your romantic relationships, your friends, your favorite movies, books, and music, and virtually every single thing on earth that you like. While you may have spent time creating the best digital version of yourself others can view and make snap judgments about, in day-to-day real life, *you* are your walking, talking profile. With all that can be accomplished online, sometimes it's easy to forget a great big world is out there, which can be seen and touched. Just like your online persona is representative of you, you are the physical representation of that persona. Try your best to look at your e-profile without bias. You'll get a good sense of who you are currently telling the world you want to be.

The ads you are drawn to, the places where you enjoy shopping, your favorite films, books, and music, and even your online profiles have hopefully helped paint a clearer picture of who you are. Now it's time to figure out "What do I want to say?"

In step 2, when we discussed first impressions and dressing for your day, we posed two key questions. First, am I comfortable? Second, what word or sentence am I trying to convey? Here is where we'll fine-tune the answers. Taking into account your goals will help you really understand your comfort, aside from the obvious physical aspect, as well as what word, sentence, or message you are sending via your style.

When it comes to comfort, depending on your objective, it isn't only about fit—making sure your clothes and shoes are the right size. It's also about what's appropriate to the setting of your day. Will the setting be cold or hot, windy or rainy? If you're spending a day at the beach with family or friends, you'll want to plan accordingly and wear something light and airy, but also bring an extra cover-up to protect you from the sun. If you're going to an outdoor cocktail party, bring a chic shawl or sweater and toss an extra umbrella in the car, just in case. If you aren't prepared for the elements, you'll be uncomfortable. Trust me. I know we've all suffered for fashion, but if you're freezing, sunburned, or soaked, the only message people will hear is "I'm miserable."

"What Do I Want to Say?"

While verbal language is how we directly communicate messages, your style speak is more open to interpretation. If you're tired or hungry or happy, you might say so aloud, eliminating any confusion about what it is you're trying to convey. With style, however, if you don't know what you're communicating, the world may get the wrong message. So in order to break down what your style is saying, you first have to consider your short- and long-term goals. Your short-term goals change daily. Today you may have a work meeting, where your goal is to win new business; tomorrow you may have your daughter's soccer game, and your objectives are to remember to wash her uniform and get everyone to and from the game safely. While your outfit choices for each of these days will likely be very different, your individual brand stays the same—it's the message that changes. Long-term goals are often accomplished slowly over the course of achieving many daily, short-term goals. If you're working toward a work promotion, trying to meet someone special, or simply hoping to have better control of your image, understanding your brand and clarifying your style speak will help you achieve it.

Aside from the setting, consider the occasion when thinking about your comfort. A common concern for many is being over- or underdressed for an event. While it's relatively easy to decipher what's appropriate for attending church versus going dancing, there is a lot of gray area in between. For these events, you should focus less on conforming to what other people may expect of you (which often leads to discomfort when you wear something that isn't *you*) and more on being respectful while also representing your unique spirit. For example, think about attending a wedding where friends and family mix. This scenario is a common style challenge for many because it requires a little more thought and balance than other situations. The purpose of the occasion is to celebrate the bride and groom, not find a date or network (although if either of those things happen organically, fantastic!). So your primary goal is to demonstrate that you care about this special moment in someone's life and put effort into your appearance. In fact, in situations like these, what you're not saying can be just as powerful as what you are. If you aren't communicating respect, the lack thereof is a pretty powerful message people in attendance, especially the bride and groom, will hear. This isn't to say that you don't also want to be the best version of yourself; you just don't want to pull focus. Wearing a low-cut or too-tight dress may offend those who want the occasion to be reverent, and arriving in something dirty or worn, or having paid minimal attention to your hair or makeup, might show a lack of interest. It's about balance, and if you're considerate of the occasion and confident in your attire, you eliminate the need to worry about whether you're over- or underdressed.

Understanding your goals will also help you better construct the word or sentence you wish to convey. In an instance when your goal is specific and timely, this adjective or phrase can go a long way toward ensuring that your style speak is helping you accomplish it (e.g., the bank appointment example from step 2, when the phrase conjured was "financially responsible"). When you have mentally highlighted a distinct goal and corresponding adjective like this, planning an outfit for unique occasions becomes much easier. Most days, however, when nothing remarkable or unusual is planned,

Worthwhile Words

I have three go-to adjectives that help me decide what to wear depending on my daily goals. Feel free to borrow mine or come up with your own:

STRIKING . . . is what I envision for those moments when my goal is to stand out, be memorable, or get noticed. I think *striking* when I'm prepping for a red-carpet appearance, a presentation, or a party. Simply shifting my mind to focus on this word helps me decide if my style choice is saying what I want it to.

CHIC . . . is a word I concentrate on when my goal is to feel graceful and stylish without being flashy. When the situation is not about calling attention to myself, I aim to embody chic, which for me implies a modern twist on a classic.

INVITING . . . is for those occasions when my goal is to engage. Whether personally or professionally, when I want to be emotionally close with others and connect with them, I strive to send out an inviting message. I think of these as moments when I socialize with my girlfriends or spend time with my family members or a significant other.

Having these go-to words has worked for me. Keeping a list of commonly used adjectives and goals in mind will help you better carve out your intentions and your style speak.

Image Is Everything

I often find that celebrity examples are particularly helpful and powerful, because not only are these people extremely aware of and (usually) in control of their personal brands, but we, the public, are ultimately in charge of how their brands are perceived. Growing up in Los Angeles, I had many friends and social acquaintances who were part of the Hollywood scene. Early in my career, I wrote an advice column for a teen magazine and would occasionally interview some of my famous friends to get their insights into style and self-esteem. From Pink to Jessica Simpson to Britney Spears, each of these women had a very specific brand and a style they communicated to the world (and in these cases it really was the whole world watching and listening to them). Alecia Moore, the artist known to millions as "Pink," in particular, has always been an inspiration to me. When she hit the music scene, people didn't know how to react. She was often ridiculed for her clothes, her hair, and her outgoing I-don't-give-a-sh*t attitude. I admired her courage to be herself among the sea of female pop stars at the time. When she introduced herself, *everyone* had a reaction. Her overall style may still be considered extreme, but that's who she is. She's a strong, fiercely independent woman, and these attributes shine through in everything from her music to her outfit choices and accessories to her various hair colors and tattoos.

Jennifer Aniston is another strong celebrity example of effective style speak and branding, but from a completely different perspective. While Pink employs an outward, animated approach, Jennifer has always been much more subtle. From casual to classic, she has found a way to brand the effortless, American-girl look, and in some ways has become a style icon just by being the girl next door. She has gone from wildly successful television actor to leading lady to national superstar whose every move is captured in magazines, yet her laid-back style remains consistent. It's this congruency between the fun-loving woman we all wanted to hang out with on *Friends* and the approachable style she continues to convey that keeps her one of America's sweethearts.

Pink and Jennifer are two great examples of celebrities whose styles reinforce their personalities and contribute to the over-all strength of their brands. With these women, what you see is what you get. But there are plenty of examples of what happens when the opposite occurs. One of the sweetest people I've ever had the privilege to get to know is Britney Spears. To those close to her, Britney has always been an innocent, bubbly Southern girl with a huge talent. When you think about Britney now, what has been so controversial about her stems from the incongruence be-tween her personality and her public persona. We immediately fell in love with the squeaky-clean pop star when she first jumped onto the scene, but everything blew up when we started to see her mature and embrace her sexier side. Her eventual meltdown came because the image she was being asked to portray to the world wasn't authentic to who she was. The Britney I knew would have had no problem walking barefoot into a gas station in her hometown, wearing ripped jeans shorts and no makeup every day. That's who she is. But the media didn't accept these behaviors. This distrust not only caused controversy on the outside but, on a personal level, also caused her a lot of turmoil.

Whether you're a celebrity or not, everyone you interact with is listening to your style. If it conflicts with your true self, your intentions run the risk of being misinterpreted, which can have confusing and unintended results. When you project an image and message that clearly reinforce who you are, you help clarify your goals and complement your personality. It's when you radiate this type of confidence and authenticity that people can't help but no-tice and react to you.

your goals, and therefore the words or sentences you want to express, are less specific. It's because of these days (most days) that I encourage you to come up with a few goals and corresponding adjectives to strengthen your style speak on a daily basis.

The bottom line is that having a firm grasp on who you are and what you want to say allows you take control of your style speak, highlight your personal brand, and achieve your goals. My role is to help you evaluate your image, because while you may not be able to control how others perceive you, you can and should take charge of the message you are sending out. And as it is said, "Luck is when preparation meets opportunity." I am here to help you prep, so you can attract your own opportunities and all the "luck" that follows.

ADVERTISE ACCURATELY

At this point, you are well on your way toward purposefully speaking your own style. You have a much better understanding about who you are and what you want to say. The only thing left between you and your effective, accurate style speak is mastering the art of self-endorsement. Sure, you know what you have to offer the world, but how do you entice the world to listen? How are you going to best promote *you*? Consumer brands are promoted via advertising, one of the most powerful industries in the world. In 2011 alone the United States spent $144 billion on advertising (according to data released by Kantar Media), so obviously the way a product looks and how it is positioned is extremely important to these brands and worth investing in. The same goes for you. While you're now the proud owner of your own brand, are you proactively creating your advertising messages? What do you want other people to know about you? Be your own one-person PR department and decide what your tagline or sixty-second commercial is going to be.

Think about sixty seconds: the moments of missed opportunity in life when you wish you had said this or done that. Why not have a go-to mantra or theme song? (Who remembers the popular TV show from the nineties *Ally McBeal*? Kids, Google it.) Then, when that moment of opportunity presents itself (e.g., when a sexy stranger on the street asks you a question or you find yourself in the elevator with the head of your department), you'll be better prepared to *carpe diem*. For me, whenever I need a little extra confidence boost, I borrow inspiration from the song "There She Goes" by Babyface, featuring Pharrell. The upbeat tempo combined with lyrics like "Her style, her mind, compares to nothing on this earth . . . only God knows what she's worth" and "She's incredible . . . her walk, her talk, her way, her savoir faire" give me a little extra push.

So let's build a personal advertising plan that showcases the authentic you. Since all good promotional campaigns follow certain guidelines to achieve success, I've taken inspiration from some of the best in the biz to help you *identify* your unique assets, *target* your message, *display* your best features, and then *pay attention* to feedback.

Identify: Highlight Your Assets

In the business world, the first step in creating a promotional campaign is to identify your unique selling proposition, or USP. Simply put, it's the process of uncovering what differentiates your product—in this case *you*—from others. Years ago, when I was first trying to carve out my own place in the entertainment world, a talent agent suggested I write down all my thoughts on my "brand." Doing so not only helped me better articulate my professional goals, but also helped me understand how I could uniquely position myself. She referred to this as brand homework, and at the time I remember thinking "Everyone should do this!" To better discover the unique things that make you stand out in the world, answer the following questions. I've included a few sample answers to help guide you:

WHAT FIVE ADJECTIVES BEST DESCRIBE MY PERSONALITY?

(Different, fresh, positive, inventive, original, modern, contemporary, accessible, warm, practical, genuine, honest, charming, caring, sensitive, sweet, confident, etc.)

WHAT ARE MY STRENGTHS AND SKILLS?

(I'm a great cook, I know how to throw a beautiful party, I'm a good listener, I speak many different languages, etc.)

WHAT DO PEOPLE THINK OF ME?
(LIST THREE TO FIVE WORDS.)

(Strong, motivated, fun, etc.)

_____

_____

WHAT AM I PASSIONATE ABOUT?
WHAT ARE MY HOBBIES? INTERESTS?

(What do you like to do in your free time? Here, I like to think about the old career advice I got in high school and college: "What would you want to do even if you weren't getting paid?" Whether you jog, scrapbook, sew, or play video games, write it down.)

_____

_____

_____

WHAT DO I DO? AND HOW DOES IT
AFFECT OTHERS OR ADD VALUE?

(This can be a profession or a larger calling. For example: I'm a nurse. I make people feel safe and comforted. I encourage people to smile and aim to make everyone in my life look on the bright side of things. At work, I use my knowledge of medicine to help people feel comfortable and get healthy. At home, I use the bedside manner I've developed over the years to resolve conflicts between family and friends.)

_____

_____

_____

WHO DO YOU IDENTIFY WITH?

(Maybe you identify with Jane Austen's character Emma, or your best friend, or Cher. Whoever it is, write his or her name down and include why.)

_____

_____

_____

I have done an extensive version of this exercise as well, and it was helpful for me to recognize the things about myself I think are distinct. Specifically, after answering these questions, I realized how my background in psychology is linked to my passion for style and part of the reason I have worked hard to share my philosophy with others. Consider your responses. Can you come up with a few things you feel set you apart from everyone else? Keep these in mind the next time you shop or interact in social settings. If you feel your sense of humor, your profession, or your unique skills or talents identify you as a person, make sure you call these things out and play them up so others can appreciate them about you as well. You want to make sure you use your energies in the best ways possible. Whether it's highlighting what you're good at or investing in other areas to become well rounded, there is much to be gained from taking this inventory.

Target: Know Your Audience

To ensure that your style speak is helping you achieve your desired results, you have to reach the right people in the first place. So the next step is to know your audience. What's your life like? Who do you interact with the most? What situations do you encounter in a typical day? We are diverse and complicated beings, so this answer can and will vary greatly from person to person. If you're a twenty-two-year-old kindergarten teacher in the suburbs, your audience throughout most of the day will be vastly different from that of a forty-five-year-old tattoo artist in a big city. As we've discussed, considering your daily objectives is important when crafting your style messages, but it's also essential to pinpoint the people who will help you achieve them. You want to be sure your message is really connecting with those around you and doing so in a meaningful way. A new kindergarten teacher might want to wear brighter colors, choose outfits that convey warmth and trust, and should probably leave the platform heels in her car for later, whereas a tattoo artist should feel motivated to express her personality at work, with accents that hint at her unique interests. In knowing your audience, you can help use your personal image to better communicate with the people in your life.

This is not to say you should adjust your style speak to fit other people's expectations. While you may not realize it, you have chosen your audience as a result of the decisions you've made and the paths you've taken so far in your life. The exchange that occurs every day between you and others is at least partially of your own doing; when it comes to your end of the communication, being 100 percent self-sacrificing (telling them only what they want to hear) or 100 percent self-serving (telling them only what you want to say) isn't productive. You have to factor in your intentions along with who is listening in order to create the most successful ad plan.

Display: Know What You're Packaging

Presentation is everything. So another important element to factor into your overall nonverbal PR plan is your packaging—how you display your message. While the biggest element of this might fall to fashion, don't neglect all the others that contribute to your total look, from your accessories to hairstyles to beauty-product choices and beyond.

How do you feel when you see a beautifully wrapped gift? Corporations spend enormous amounts of time, energy, and money every year coming up with packaging concepts that will attract and stimulate consumers to purchase their products. So what sort of investment are you making in your packaging? Knowing yourself and your unique style speak will take you only so far if you throw an old overcoat over your cute outfit or neglect to comb your hair, inevitably muzzling your message before you walk out the door. In fact, your packaging is so important that the entire second half of this book is devoted to the tools that will help you create your best visual self. Yet your overall style package is the combined total of what can be seen *and* unseen. You have to know who you are, have confidence in yourself, and allow your body language to reinforce your message and intentions. Paying attention to details and adding those little extras that make you *you*—anything from your signature scent, which lingers when you leave the room, to always remembering the birthdays of friends and coworkers—create your overall packaging theme. It's important to think about how you present yourself to those you interact with so you can make sure you're strengthening rather than weakening your message.

Pay Attention: Listen to Feedback

Just like in the consumer advertising world, there are ways to measure the success of your personal advertising plan. It's all about listening to feedback. In the beginning of this step we discussed how communication is a two-way street, with one person sending out a message and another perceiving it. It's important to note that this process continues back and forth like a tennis match. You send a message, someone perceives it and returns a message related to that perception. You then perceive that person's message and the process continues. We've now spent time carefully crafting who you are, what you want to say, and how to begin saying it. The final test is to listen to how people are perceiving you. Are you:

- delivering your message clearly?
- confirming your credibility or authenticity?
- connecting to your audience?
- attracting loyalty?

The best way to tell if your personal advertising plan is working is to pay attention to these goals. When you notice people are reacting to who you are (perhaps complimenting your appearance or trusting you with more responsibility at work) and responding to you positively, they are hearing your style speak. If not, you may need to think about and adjust one or more of your variables. (Are you conscious of your short- and long-term goals? Are you comfortable? Are you taking your audience into account?) Additionally, make sure you're not just hearing what you want to.

Sometimes it's hard to hear things about ourselves that aren't fantastic, but it's all part of learning, growing, and becoming the best possible version of you.

THE EVOLUTION OF STYLE SPEAK

At this point I hope you feel extremely comfortable with the idea of style speak and are ready to start wearing your carefully crafted language to your advantage. But let me leave you with one last important note. Your style is extremely personal and constantly evolving. It's a fluid process of discovery, influenced by your situations as well as your personal evolution. Similar to your taste in foods, your favorite types of music, and the television shows you watch on a regular basis, your style sensibilities will change over the years. I don't know about you, but I'm a much different person today than I was ten, fifteen, and twenty years ago. So remember that discovering your style is a journey, not a destination.

As the style editor for a morning news program, I have the opportunity to discuss style with women of all ages. From helping teenagers choose the perfect prom dresses to making maternity wear more fashionable for first-time moms to translating trends for seniors, I have seen a lot over the years, and I know firsthand how personal brands and subsequent style speak can change.

Think about it. Your teen years are all about experimentation. It's a time when you're overwhelmed with choices and decisions, and when you first start to develop your style sensibilities. Your twenties are a time of exploration. You may move away from your childhood home, start a career, live alone for the first time, or experience your first serious relationship. This is a time to discover what you like and don't like (with limited influence from others who may have affected you in the past, including family and school friends).

In your thirties you likely gain more of a foundation and really establish yourself in the life you began cultivating in your twenties. Perhaps you invest in more statement pieces, or you've begun to neglect your style to focus more on marriage or children. If you're a working gal, it's likely during these years that you'll devote more time to your career, so developing a unique style that works for your professional life as well as your personal one is important.

Your forties are a great time to take mental (and physical) inventory of your stuff and your style. Probably you've been amassing items from previous years—maybe things you've held on to for emotional reasons or because you're anticipating old trends will come back around. This time period is when you can investigate what's really working for you, what's worth holding on to, and what can be purged. It's also a great time to evaluate current trends and look into incorporating the ones you like into your current style.

Your fifties and sixties are wonderful for fashion. Remember that popular country song by Wade Hayes titled "Old Enough to Know Better"? That line, "I'm old enough to know better but I'm still too young to care," reminds me of the fashionable women I know in their fifties and sixties. You've seen trends come and go, probably tried a number of different hairstyles and makeup brands, and learned a thing or two about who you are and what works best for you. I love taking advice from seasoned women in my life who have reached this age and have invaluable insights to share about style. But the reverse is true as well. This is a great time to take cues from what the younger generations are interested in. I love seeing sophisticated women surprise me with a bold streak of color in their hair, platform pumps, or a funky twist on a menswear-inspired look.

The same goes for the seventy-plus set. My friend Ari Seth Cohen's blog (and book) *Advanced Style* highlights an amazing group of women over seventy who embody the idea of true style speak in ways I feel we could all learn from. They demonstrate that it's not about numbers—age, weight, price, etc.—but about letting go and allowing yourself to embrace your individuality. While many of us fear aging, when I spoke to hundred-year-old Ruth, who does Pilates every week and wears lipstick even when she goes to the hospital because she never knows who she's going to meet, and ninety-two-year-old Ilona, who makes her own false eyelashes and sings in cabaret shows, they both told me the same thing: they wish they had been as self-assured in their own skins earlier in life. The ease and confidence with which these women express themselves are nothing short of awe inducing. They break conventional fashion "rules," take chances, and make no apologies for who they are. They have developed loud, clear, and beautiful versions of individual style speak and are very aware of their messages. They are living examples of how style truly is self-expression and that, in the words of Ann Moore (former CEO of Time, Inc.), it's important to "follow your compass, not your clock."

If you feel like you're looking at all the nuts and bolts lying on the floor and are overwhelmed by how to build the dresser, pause to understand that it's an accomplishment in itself to have answered the questions posed in this step. Knowing who you are and what you want to say—both of which can change throughout your life—is a big undertaking. But this food for thought will help guide you in developing your own style, from deciding between a wedge and a stiletto, or a blazer and a cardigan. After all, you have to know *who* you're dressing before you can successfully dress her. Understanding what your brand is, how to communicate it via style speak, and how to effectively advertise yourself all comprise the foundation from which you can begin to match your outside to your inside.

But before we get there, I want to make sure you both know your own worth and are ready to commit to the process.

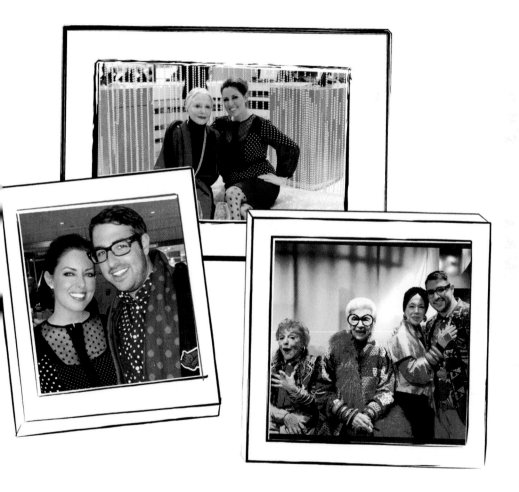

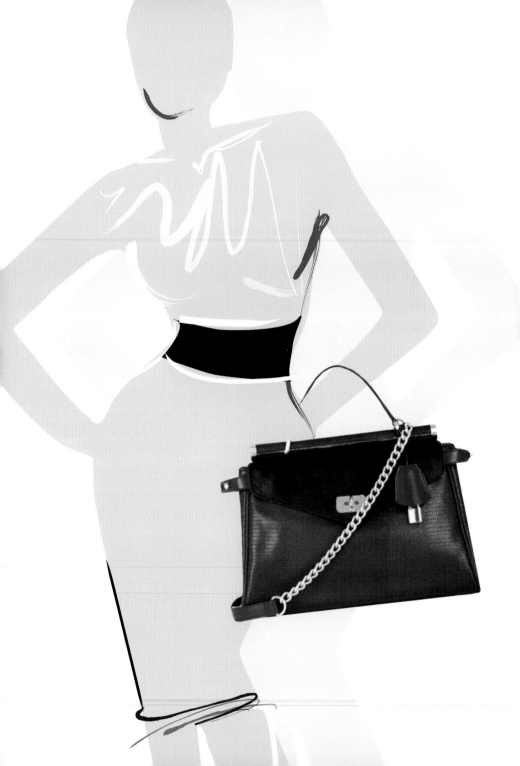

KNOW YOUR WORTH

Prioritize Yourself

"Because I'm worth it," said Ilon Specht. This famous line is not only one of my all-time favorite beauty-brand slogans, but also, whether you're aware of it or not, the reason you picked up this book in the first place. Understanding the importance of your own reflection, the power of your body language, and how to harness your style speak won't add up to much if you don't care enough about yourself to put these tools into practice.

In 1973, when twenty-three-year-old female Ilon Specht coined this phrase, men were still the primary audience for advertisers, making this women-centric campaign somewhat controversial. (Women are worth it? Who knew?!) But the notion caught fire and now, decades later, commercials and print ads are still declaring to you that you're worth it. But how often do you say it to yourself? Probably not often enough. As women, we are blessed with the instinct to want to put others before ourselves. Many of us tend to think of the wants and needs of our children, spouses, siblings, and even friends before we pause to pay any leftover attention to ourselves. But you're more than worth the time and energy it takes to invest in being your best. In fact, it's when you feel most worthy that you're better able to confidently share your skills, talents, and energy with others.

Your style is how you communicate to the world. It's your self-expression, how people perceive you, how you visually articulate who you are as well as your interests and goals, and it can be one of your greatest sources of self-confidence. Style is significant enough for celebrities, dignitaries, and CEOs to regularly hire experts just to help them prep and plan how to present themselves. However, acknowledging that most mortals don't have this luxury, style is sadly one of the first things sacrificed in order to focus on other "more important" elements of life.

I have heard too often and from too many women that they just don't have the time to focus on fashion or go shopping. Sure, in some extreme cases this may be true. But in others, it may be a way to avoid negative feelings about yourself. For example, if you're unhappy with your weight, chances are you don't enjoy trying on new clothes in a public fitting room. Never mind the unflattering overhead lights or shared mirror space; the emotional task of acknowledging your body image can leave you feeling discouraged. Here's where the professional friend (and maybe annoying cheerleader) in me tells you that you shouldn't give up. Never, ever, ever give up on you. Finding something to wear that makes you feel beautiful is a likely possibility, but more important, do you really want to ignore what you're unhappy about? If you aren't feeling your best and you shy away from presenting your best self, you're actually adding another layer to your insecurity, which further affects your true style. Awareness offers you an opportunity to make a change.

Confidence is the key to unlocking your inner worth so you can confront any issues you may be avoiding.

> Never, ever, ever give up on you.

CORE CONFIDENCE

If you're simply concerned with looking like the celebrity du jour on the cover of *Vanity Fair*, you'll never win. But if you're reading this book because you want to look in the mirror and think you *deserve* to be on the cover of that magazine, then you're already ahead in the game. I know being completely self-assured is sometimes easier said than done, but you'll have to take a leap of faith with me here. I believe most things in life are accomplished as a direct result of how much confidence you approach them with. In many cases, even more than your actual skill, qualifications, or the quality of your work, your confidence in what you're doing, saying, or wearing will make you more likely to succeed. Have you ever seen a woman walking down the street, head held high, in something you would never have the guts to wear? Sure you have. It could've been a backless dress, a bright orange muumuu, a leopard-print jumpsuit, or a fascinator or fanciful hat, but whatever it was, my question to you is why did you feel you couldn't wear what she did? With the exception of any physical or professional restraints, the answer likely has a lot to do with your overall confidence.

So often we're afraid people will find out we're a fraud. We fear our lover will find out we're not sexy. We fear our colleagues will discover we're not smart. We fear our friends will uncover that we're not happy. This fear is based on the fact that we don't think we're any of these things. Or perhaps we're afraid to succeed. In a world obsessed with a "perfect" outside, why wouldn't we be afraid to express the inside? Our worst fears are that we won't be good enough, lovable, or worthy. In other words, what if we aren't perfect? The truth is the world won't crumble and we won't be banned from our villages because of our nonphysical imperfections any more than for our physical ones.

> Our worst fears are that we won't be good enough, lovable, or worthy. In other words, what if we aren't perfect?

In order to foster a strong sense of confidence you have to overcome these fears and take a few risks. In fact, the best way to build up your self-esteem is by putting yourself out there and accepting the responses, good or bad. This attitude is how you build what I like to call "core confidence." Core confidence is the genuine, authentic poise that comes from placing value in you and in your unique qualities and characteristics. When you emanate core confidence, it doesn't matter if some of the reactions you get from the world are negative, because you believe in yourself. At the end of the day, you are the only critic that matters.

Despite knowing that the key to worth is confidence, it's not exactly helpful to simply say "be confident" or "believe in yourself" and leave it at that. You have to take a look at what you value in order to determine where your confidence is coming from.

INTRINSIC VERSUS EXTRINSIC VALUE

What do you value? Where does your self-esteem come from? Since style is self-expression, it's important to build your sense of self-worth on a strong foundation rather than on fleeting physical attributes or external factors. This is the difference between intrinsic self-esteem and extrinsic self-esteem. So often we've seen friends, loved ones, and even ourselves assign importance to relationships, material possessions, and status symbols. We've all done it, and I am no exception. During college I even transferred to an out-of-state school with my boyfriend because his football career dominated our relationship. Although my tuition fees dramatically increased, I thought making that sacrifice was expected of "the quarterback's

INTRINSIC WORTH VERSUS EXTRINSIC WORTH

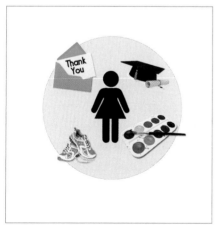 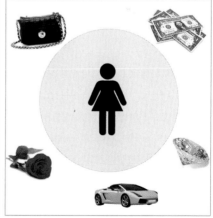

girlfriend." I ceased being myself in favor of being his girlfriend. You probably know someone who has made a similar decision, trying to stay connected to the "right" friends or forgoing her career or putting her passion on hold to be "the doctor's wife" or something similar. While there is absolutely nothing wrong with taking pride in your significant other's accomplishments, this is not where you should be sourcing your self-worth. Nor should you fall victim to assigning value to other extrinsic things, be it your job, a luxury car, a designer handbag, or an expensive home in a desired neighborhood. The truth is, the boyfriend can break up with you, you can lose your job, and the car can get totaled. If the basis of your self-esteem is temporary, or controlled by factors beyond your reach, it will be difficult to withstand the challenges life will surely throw at you. And this breeds insecurity, which can be a woman's biggest nemesis. So don't allow others to tell you who you are or what you're worth. Equating all your inner value with these things is akin to building a house of cards; it easily tumbles.

Intrinsic self-esteem, on the other hand, is something that can never be taken away from you. Your accomplishments, character traits, unique qualities, and skills will still be with you no matter what else happens in life. It's these things you should look to when you need to reach into your confidence reserves. I think of the concept of DIY whenever I speak to others about self-esteem, because I feel it's in creation that we, as people, hold a lot of integrity. If you're good at sewing, painting, or crafting, or if you aren't a DIY gal at all but can make a delicious meal, or you never cook but always know the best delivery places and the exact right time to call—anything you're uniquely good at and take pride in can be a place from which you get your self-confidence.

What intrinsic qualities and talents do you place your value in?

_____

_____

_____

_____

_____

_____

_____

It can be as simple as common courtesy. I once was invited to attend a dinner hosted by shoe designer Stuart Weitzman and invited my friend JL to come along. JL is the kind of thoughtful person who pays attention to detail, and she had once heard that Mr. Weitzman loved Mallomars. Although she had never met him in person, she arrived with an array of the chocolate-coated marshmallow treats as a gift for the host. Where many other people would have gone the classic wine route or in some cases not brought a gift at all, JL went that little extra step. This consideration is an extension of her style and something she can be proud of.

All these intangible elements are extensions of style. So often when people hear the word "style" they immediately think "fashion." But fashion is an external thing, not a way to identify yourself, whereas style is about being whole and balanced. As the iconic former *Vogue* editor Edna Woolman Chase once said, "Fashion can be bought. Style one must possess."

The most stylish people I know emanate from the inside out a core confidence and comfort in their own skin. It's important to note that some of the most stylish people in history weren't simply the prettiest or the wealthiest. Confidence is contagious, and the people I respect most are those who are willing and able to inspire others by simply being themselves. When you nurture your gifts, talents, and education—not cars, accessories, or job titles—you will be self-sufficient, not codependent. And when you take the time to proudly display your intrinsic qualities, instead of going with the grain and meeting the expected minimum, that's when you will be able to define yourself and embrace that definition. You will be secure and *own* your sense of worth, instead of just renting it.

> "Fashion can be bought. Style one must possess."
>
> —Edna Woolman Chase

TIME FOR TLC

In addition to sourcing your confidence intrinsically, another way to ensure you're investing in your own worth is by taking care of yourself. Think about why you care for a possession. It's because you value it. If you have a nice handbag, you are far less likely to put it on the floor or carelessly toss it into your car than you are an older, beat-up sack you don't care as much about. If you don't value yourself, or you beat yourself up, why would you want to take care of your physical and emotional well-being? I'm not demanding that

Bobbie's Stress Busters

Some very simple pampering can go a long way. To ensure that you're taking proper care of yourself, try to remember these stress busters.

SMILE: Smiling has more benefits than you may know. If you're feeling down, it can trick your body into feeling happier by releasing more endorphins. It can boost your immune system. It's even said that smiling can make you look younger!

SIP: Water is nature's most rejuvenating resource. When I sip water throughout the day, I tend to eat healthier and feel more alert. Plus, it's fantastic for your skin, nails, and hair.

SOAK: Bubbles or no bubbles, melt away stress in the bathtub to recharge your muscles and your mind.

SLEEP: There is no substitute for a good night's rest. Whenever possible, I try to make sure I'm getting a full eight hours, even if it means missing a favorite TV show from time to time.

STRETCH: As we age, our muscles tighten. Stretching reduces tension, increases blood flow, and gives you more energy throughout the day.

SOCIALIZE: We are social creatures, so reach out and call someone. Join a book club or an exercise class, or take a wine-tasting course. It's healthy to break up your routine and mingle with new people.

STOP: And smell the roses or gush over an adorable baby or puppy on the street. Allow yourself to take time out and appreciate the little things every once in a while.

you love everything about your current state, including your body, your finances, your job, and all your relationships with every single person in your life. (Although, if you do, congratulations and please e-mail me your secrets.) What I am suggesting is that you pay attention to yourself. Are you eating healthy, exercising, avoiding sun damage, making sure you don't drink to excess? Are you setting time aside just for you? Do you ever go for walks simply to breathe the air and clear your head? When was the last time you danced? Some of these may sound silly, but they are all things many of us forget to do regularly, and they can affect our overall self-value. In the same way you wouldn't buy a new dress and then throw it on the floor of your closet in a crumpled pile, take pride in yourself and show yourself some TLC.

I fully acknowledge that taking care of one's self requires time and energy. We can't live at a spa or take month-long vacations from life in order to recharge. But remember, input equals output; you can't expect the results you want in life if you're not willing to put forth any effort. Furthermore, everything comes at a cost, so invest in yourself and in the things that bring you happiness. It doesn't have to be the newest designer jeans or sunglasses. It could be finding a new song to download, buying a pretty candle just because, splurging on a slice of cake from the best bakery in town, scooping up some fresh flowers, or convincing your friends to plan a girlfriend getaway. Just make sure you aren't skimping when it comes to your own happiness.

Don't be afraid to spend time on yourself. I'm always perplexed by those who say "Why make the bed since no one else is here to notice?" or "I'm not going to go to the trouble to cook a meal just for myself." Each morning I make my bed because I like the way it looks. I wash my dishes after a meal rather than allowing them to pile up in the sink because it bothers me to have unsightly pots and pans cluttering up my kitchen. I enjoy cooking myself a delicious meal *because* it's just me, not *although* it's just me. Taking care of and investing time in yourself are the ways in which you demonstrate self-respect and self-worth.

While you make these investments, it's also imperative that you not put any unnecessary pressure on yourself. This boils down to acceptance.

ACCEPTANCE

Before you can love your style, you have to love yourself. And part of knowing your own worth is accepting yourself. If you're waiting until the day when your life is perfect to truly feel worthy, it might be a long wait. You are worthy right now, as is. When you recognize that there are some things in life you can control and some you can't, you are able to shift your focus to only those that are in your power. This acceptance is what will make you feel good enough, strong enough, and prepared to make positive changes.

It's human to have bad days and to judge ourselves, but when we do this, it's usually because we are comparing ourselves to others. In general, but particularly when it comes to style, this can be unhealthy, especially considering today's impossible beauty standards based on supermodels and airbrushing. It's essential to create your own standards, so you don't end up tirelessly pursuing or envious of an ideal that doesn't really exist in the first place. Don't chase the unicorn. Negative feelings are red flags, so pay attention if you're feeling envious or having a why-not-me moment. In case you're perfect, here is a list of things people commonly get jealous of: other people's jobs, other people's money (i.e., other people's trust funds or parents' trust funds), other people's bodies (big boobs, flawless skin, long legs, flat stomachs, etc.), other people's friends or relationships, other people's homes or cars, other people's clothes or accessories, other people's number of Twitter followers, other people's knowledge of current events, music, or fine wines, other people's joke-telling abilities—the list goes on and on. Accept yourself and stop comparing. Work with what you have to create your ideal you, instead of a mix-and-match version of other people.

Years ago I was feeling sorry for myself, and a friend wisely said to me, "When you think the grass is greener, it's time to water your own." It was as if someone turned on the lights. Ever since, this one quote has offered me an invaluable perspective for so many situations, and I have adopted it as my personal mantra.

> "When you think the grass is greener, it's time to water your own."

It was reinforced not long ago while I was having lunch with a few female acquaintances at a sidewalk café. A woman around our age walked by wearing a pair of tight running pants and a sports bra, presumably on her way to the gym. After she passed, one of the girls I was lunching with said aloud, "Can you believe her? She must really need attention." The other women agreed, quick to tear down this stranger simply because she was confident enough to show off a body she had clearly worked for. As women, many of us are sadly programmed to compete with and feel jealous of other women, when we should want to support our fellow females and allow their successes to inspire us to work on ourselves. While these women criticized another's self-expression, I was reminded of my friend's quote and of how, when you know your own worth and accept yourself, you are far less likely to want to diminish someone else.

Make a list of all the things in your life you wish were different. (You can use the box below.) Then take that list and highlight just those items you feel confident you can change. You have just taken

Improvement items:

1. _____

_____

2. _____

_____

3. _____

_____

4. _____

_____

5. _____

_____

the first step toward acceptance. I'm not saying to give up on improving anything you don't have complete control over, but tackle the can-do ones first and allow yourself to accept the rest—at least until after you've achieved your can-do list. Then you can revisit and reassess the other original items. Your style should always be on your can-do list. When you've filtered out any other hurdles and learned to accept what you cannot change, the process gets easier.

PEOPLE ARE PRESENTS

In step 3 I shared the importance of paying attention to your packaging, but this can be a tall order if you don't feel worthy enough to invest in it, and I don't mean just monetarily. A long time ago, I was introduced to the notion that people are presents—we all walk around in our unique wrapping, attracting others to want to know more about what's inside. If someone was to hand you a gift wrapped in bright, beautiful paper adorned with ribbons and another wrapped haphazardly in old newspaper, which one would you be more excited to open? The way you dress is your wrapping. It's intended to be the best representation of who you are and what's inside you, and to attract those who want to get to know you better.

This can get tricky if you shift the focus from what's inside (your gift) to emphasize only your outside wrapping. When this happens, you lose sight of *you* and risk becoming a walking billboard for the idea someone else has of you, which could be your mother's notion of how you should dress, your husband's, a friend's, or the latest seasonal ad campaign. If you're obsessed with wearing only the hottest labels, you may attract someone's attention with your flashy designer duds, but what will he or she see when you hang your Chanel jacket up in the closet? Don't get me wrong; I love designer pieces just as much as the next gal and have definitely squealed with delight over a handbag or had my spirits lifted by a pair of stilettos from time to time. I've seen firsthand that money looks good on many a person. But money, and the high-priced fashion and resources it provides, should simply amplify who you were to start with. So please understand that I'm not dissing luxury labels or designer accessories. I'm simply saying to use them as a tool, not a crutch. By the same token, why spend time and money having a beautifully manicured front lawn if the inside of your house is a disaster area? If your packaging is a true reflection of who you are, when the attention shifts from your fashion to your inner self, the transition will be seamless.

The reverse of putting too much emphasis on ornate packaging can be an equally tricky problem, to not pay *enough* attention to your wrapping. Going back to the two differently packaged gifts, while the extravagant wrapping may have initially attracted you, you didn't know what was inside and risked opening up a box containing a lump of coal, whereas the simple newspaper-wrapped box could have contained a beautiful scarf or a diamond necklace. This sort of misrepresentation happens all the time with style. If you aren't displaying the best, most polished version of yourself, people will assume less than the best about you. Spend the time and energy building your core confidence and investing in your packaging so that it suits you.

PAY IT FORWARD

Transitioning out of your daily routine and empowering yourself to feel truly worthy of a style investment might seem like a big task, namely because this kind of perspective shift is difficult to maintain.

Compliment Others

Today's culture conditions women to be afraid to show their vulnerable side. We are sadly bred to be competitive with one another, and oftentimes we favor dressing to "beat" other women over dressing for ourselves. For this style session, spend a day complimenting as many women as you can. Find honest, positive things you notice about other women and tell them. Everyone from your roommate, family member, or coworker to the grocery store clerk, waitress, or woman walking next to you on the street. Notice how they respond. I can all but guarantee that the results will instill a sense of confidence and self-empowerment in you both.

It may take an upfront expenditure of time, energy, and, in some cases, finances. Then you have to commit to ensuring that *you* stay your priority. If it seems like a lot to ask, I assure you it isn't. Let me remind you that you're worth it. However, if you feel yourself losing ground or having a day when your core confidence has suffered a blow, which we all will at one point or another, the easiest way to build yourself back up is by building someone else up.

The golden rule of treating everyone the way you would like to be treated is profound beyond measure, and there is a lot of truth to sayings like "It's better to give than to receive." The pride that comes from performing acts of selflessness is indescribable. Volunteering your time and talents to a place or cause close to your heart will result in an instantaneously renewed sense of self-worth. We all have bad days, or even weeks, and find ourselves stuck in the occasional rut. But the next time you feel like throwing yourself a pity party or adopting a woe-is-me attitude, know that one of the best ways to overcome adversity is by giving back. When you take the focus off your problem and transfer your energy to helping others, you amplify the good rather than the bad. Maintaining a perspective about the size of your problem in relation to others isn't about ignoring a root issue or diminishing your own challenges. It's simply about moving forward in a positive way. And sometimes the only way to bump up your self-esteem and achieve a positive enough attitude to tackle your own problem is to temporarily share in someone else's.

To be truly stylish, you have to believe in yourself. You must maintain a healthy sense of self-esteem, foster your own core confidence, take care of and accept yourself, then allow the qualities and traits you are most proud of to shine through in your packaging. Overall, you have to know your worth. Because when you feel worthy, other people will see you as worthy.

> "Our deepest fear is not that we are inadequate. Our deepest fear is that we are powerful beyond measure. It is our light, not our darkness, that most frightens us. We ask ourselves, who am I to be brilliant, gorgeous, talented, and fabulous? Actually, who are you not to be? You are a child of God. Your playing small does not serve the world."
>
> —quoted in a Nelson Mandela speech,
> originally written by Marianne Williamson

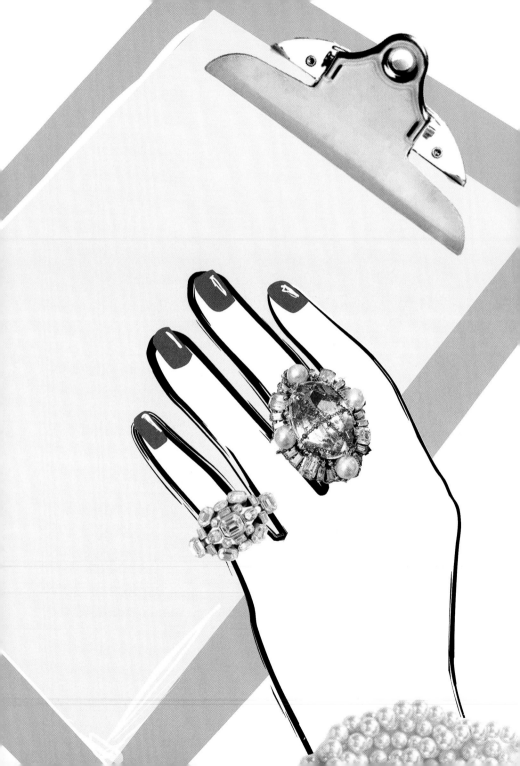

PUT A PLAN INTO PRACTICE

Make a Commitment

If there's one thing I hope you take away from everything we discussed in part I, it's that you deserve a consciously developed style reflective of how truly amazing you are. Believing in your worth, armed with a better understanding of your reflections and your body language, and taking control of your style speak to reinforce your personal brand and achieve your goals, you are just about ready to dive into part II and put it all into practice. But, like any artist about to create a beautiful work of art, you must first prep your canvas and commit to the process in order to see the best results.

You've likely heard the term "afraid to commit" a thousand times. Whether it's in the context of a serious relationship or dinner plans for next Friday, most of us have shied away from a commitment at some point in our lives. But when you commit to yourself, you should make it a priority to run full force with this promise. Devoting time to improving yourself and your life should seem like a no-brainer, but as we've discussed, with all of life's obligations we often leave ourselves for last. We allow many different obstacles to come between our want for a better style and our ability to actually go out and get it. Well, I want to help you get out of your own way and commit to finishing your style journey.

> Your style is a lifestyle choice.

Let's talk about commitment. Have you ever run a marathon? A 5K? Written a term paper? Learned a new language? Done a jigsaw puzzle? All of these things call for a commitment, and none of them can be accomplished if you quit halfway through. If you have ever tried to lose weight, you know that many of the most successful programs don't even include the word "diet" in them. Diets now have a connotation of extremes, whereas getting healthy is all about balance. It's a lifestyle change. Well, your style is a lifestyle choice. In order to take what you've learned about the importance of self-expression and really use it to your advantage, you need to commit. That's the only way you'll see lasting results. Allocating one day a week or a few days a month to consciously crafting clear style messages won't lead to a stronger brand identity any more than exercising a few days a month will lead to six-pack abs. If you do it every day, however, you're far more likely to succeed. With that in mind, you have to make yourself a priority so you can fully commit to this process.

BE YOUR OWN PRIORITY

Each one of you reading this book will have your own unique list of priorities, but one thing that should be on each and every list, regardless of your age, location, profession, or family situation, is the word "me." To make sure you stay on your list, I'm going to tackle two of the most common excuses we give to avoid prioritizing our style and ourselves.

Excuse: I don't have money.
Style Solution: Budget and be creative.

Fashion isn't free, but it doesn't have to be expensive (as I will explore in step 10, "Let's Go Shopping!"). Also, clothing is mandatory most everywhere, so you must spend money on your style regardless of your financial situation. Why not be smart about it? As in many areas of life, moderation is key. Incorporate style needs into your budget, as this will prevent you from approaching it with a feast-or-famine mentality. We've all been there in one way or another. You wait until the absolute last moment to think about a dress for that wedding or reunion because you don't want to spend the money; then you end up buying one in a panic that you don't love, and you regret it. Or maybe you allocate your shopping to one big trip a year just to get it over with, disregarding how your circumstances, tastes, and opportunities could possibly change from one month to the next. Or you're like a close friend of mine who will spend twenty dollars here and there on "cheap" trendy tidbits when what she really needs is a good winter coat that will carry her through an entire New York City winter. When you have a seasonal budget in place, it saves you from these common pitfalls.

Excuse: I don't have the time.
Style Solution: Consolidate your schedule

How much thought did you put into your outfit today? If you're like most people, you left getting dressed until the last ten minutes immediately before you had to run out the door. I call this the Daily Domino Effect. Every day many people, either knowingly or unknowingly, wait until the very last minute to throw something on before they leave their home. And every day there is an excuse. (I've been there too.) Either you're just going to work so *what does it matter*, you're toting the kids around town so *who really cares*, you're running personal errands so *no one will see you anyway*, or any of a hundred other reasons you didn't take the time to thoughtfully pick out an outfit. This cycle of doing the bare minimum tends to repeat itself, because—well, let's face it: it's easier. But knowing what you know now about how important this decision is and how it can affect everything from your mood to large life opportunities, are you starting to feel like maybe you should put a little more thought into what you're wearing on a daily basis? By allocating time to try on clothes and preplan your outfits (I call this act a "fitting") you ensure that you're confidently in control of your style speak and personal image every day.

I know most of us don't have the luxury of a fluid schedule. There's usually a set time to be in class or at work, a meeting we can't be late for, kids to drive to school, appointments to keep, etc. When this kind of buzzer looms over you, the pressure makes it hard to be creative, calm, and conscious of something that can easily be pushed to the back burner, like getting dressed. (As someone who has to regularly be ready for live television, trust me. Whether I have one or two shoes on, time's up.) But the repercussions from not taking the time to plan your outfits are great. Aside from potentially being late to your obligations, a subsequent mental effect occurs when you settle on an outfit rather than choose it. After a marathon dressing session, not only are you more likely to leave your room with most of the contents of your closet in a heap on the floor (adding one more thing to the to-do list running through your head all day), you're also more likely to feel physically uncomfortable and emotionally insecure. And as we've discussed, when you're not comfortable, physically or emotionally, you aren't putting your best self out there.

Think about it this way: you're going to spend time getting dressed regardless of how it's allocated, so doesn't it make more sense to add up those ten frazzled minutes you spend each day during a week and instead devote an hour on the weekend to a fitting? If you don't have a nine-to-five schedule, the goal is to spend the same amount of time but do it in advance, even for special occasions. Not only will you later feel good about what you're wearing, you'll also knock out the fittings faster, and because it's under your control and at your own pace, you can be more creative. Plus, it's an opportunity to realize that you may be missing a slip, some tights, or a bra you need to complete your outfit, which is helpful to know before your date is knocking on your door. So whether you're a single woman trying to juggle personal and professional pursuits or a supermom, prioritize, rearrange your routine, and find time for fittings.

By finding time for fittings, you're stacking the odds in your favor. If you love the way you look, chances are you'll feel fantastic and you'll bring that energy with you into all your daily interactions.

Style Survival 101 for Fittings

Because I've turned my passion for fashion into a career, I've gone through thousands and thousands of fittings, sometimes having to find ten to twelve outfits for one day of taping. To help you navigate the process logistically and emotionally, here are some tips I've picked up over the years.

1. FIND THE BEST TIME FOR YOU: Don't do a fitting when you first roll out of bed, or if you feel tired, sick, or crabby. Make sure you're feeling good and positive, as it will shine through in your outfits.

2. DO YOUR HAIR AND MAKEUP: Whatever your game face is, put it on before your fitting. Whether it's full makeup with lashes or just a little lip gloss, a ponytail or a styled blowout, looking and feeling finished will make a big difference. From experience I can tell you that, before having my hair and makeup done, I've tried on many a dress and tossed it into the no pile. Then, with combed hair and a little makeup, I've tried on the same dress and wondered why I didn't like it in the first place. I quickly realized it was me, not the dress, that wasn't looking so hot.

3. GET A SECOND OPINION: It's not a bad idea to have a second opinion from a friend during your fitting. It can be very helpful. Even as someone who works in the style bubble, I can't tell you how many times someone has offered me a fresh perspective (add this belt, try this brooch, etc.). It's often eye-opening to see yourself the way others see you.

There's more than one way to wear a dress, and it's fun to learn how someone else would style or accessorize your wardrobe. It's also a good excuse for a get-together. So the next time you're planning a mall trip with a girlfriend, switch the location and shop in your own closet. You can then return the favor, and you'll both get good advice and great outfit ideas.

4. MAKE IT FUN: Playing dress-up is not just for the little ones. Put on some music, pour a glass of wine, and let loose. When you enjoy the experience, you're much more likely to repeat it, and fittings can be fun!

WOULD YOU?

With the common excuses out of the way, and your name firmly on your list of priorities, we're about to begin the process of building a wardrobe reflective of you, which will help enhance your personal and professional effectiveness. Now that you know what you like, what you want to say, and all these unique and personal things about yourself, I want to ask you one more important question: Would you date you? Think about it. Whether you're married, single, or in between, really stop to consider. Would you?

Certain questions seem to cut right to the core of things. Therapists call them breakthroughs. For Oprah's disciples they are aha moments. "Would you date you?" is one of those questions for me. A while back I was helping a girlfriend get dressed for a date and we started chatting about her ideal mate. He had to be sexy,

> Would you date you?

single, smart, handsome, tall, wealthy, funny, romantic, sweet, charming, sensitive, clever, kind, generous, punctual, sincere, and of course willing to feed her bonbons in bed every night till the end of time. While he certainly sounded like a great (albeit imaginary) partner, after thinking about it, I realized that most of us want to be with the perfect person but few of us hold ourselves up to our own ideal standards. He has to have six-pack abs, yet when was the last time you were on the treadmill? You want a millionaire, yet what's your savings account balance? Coming from a good family is non-negotiable, yet could yours be guests on *Jerry Springer*?

I've found that regardless of your relationship status (and whether or not you're even interested in a partner) this simple question— Would you date you?—hits home with nearly everyone. We all want to be seen as attractive, fun, witty, intelligent, and pleasant to be around—all the traits we ourselves look for in a mate. But have you committed to being all these things?

I have since expanded on the theme: Would you hire, be friends with, live with, invest in, notice, trust you? Take a minute to really think about these questions. Maybe you are confident you would hire you, but there is no way you would ever live with you, or vice versa. In fact, most of us probably answer no to at least one of these questions.

Well, I'm here to help you commit to doing what it takes so that every day you can confidently say yes to each iteration of this question. Asking yourself these would-you questions helps to simplify the style process and aids you in measuring your progress. It highlights the areas where you're already succeeding at matching your personality to your style and makes the areas that need improvement more apparent so you can work on them. Whatever your goals

Daily First Dates

Whether you dated in the past, are currently dating, or hope to date in the future, you probably put a lot of time and effort into looking your best for a date. What if you did that every day? I'd like you to leave the house every day for a week looking the way you would if you were going on a first date, seeing your ex, going to your high school reunion, or running into your celebrity crush. For some, this may mean just putting on makeup or wearing heels. For others, it could be the whole head-to-toe look with an accessory on top. Set your goal and follow through for seven days. In a diary or on a piece of scrap paper, keep track of how this commitment influences your daily routine. For example, did your husband surprise you with flowers? Did the guy who always seems to be behind you at Starbucks pay you a compliment?

and ambitions are, using "would you" as a barometer in life will help you devote yourself to meeting them. After all, no one wants to feel undatable, unhirable, or unlovable. Nor should anyone have to.

CREATIVE VISUALIZATION

If you answered no to any of the previous would-you questions, I want you to think about what it would take for you to change your answer. Envision a version of yourself that you would date, hire, trust, be friends with, live with, etc.—a version that you are your most confident in and content with. It will be difficult to become the best you if you can't clearly see that person.

Because of this, I've found that a little creative visualization can go a long way. Shakti Gawain, in his book *Creative Visualization,* defines the concept as "the art of using mental imagery and affirmation to produce positive changes in your life." A popular practice among athletes, musicians, educators, and even those struggling with illness, it's essentially positive thinking in its most specific form. If you believe you can do, be, or accomplish something, and you focus on envisioning yourself doing, being, or accomplishing it, it's more likely you actually will.

One of the best-known studies on the practice was conducted by Russian scientists who set up four different training regimens for Olympic athletes:

- The first was composed of 100 percent physical training.

- The second was 75 percent physical training and 25 percent mental training (or creative visualization).

- The third was 50 percent physical training and 50 percent mental training (or creative visualization).

- The fourth was 25 percent physical training and 75 percent mental training (or creative visualization).

The results showed that the group who improved the most in actual performance was the fourth group, even though they did the least amount of physical training. Conversely, the first group showed the least amount of improvement, even though they exerted

Visualize Your Style

Here, we will put creative visualization into action. Imagine yourself in a scenario—at work, socializing with friends, etc. While you do this, concentrate on your goal—to be your own complete, stylish self—as this is going to further prepare you for part II. The details matter! What does your hair look like? How did you do your makeup? What are you wearing? What color is your outfit? How confident are you feeling? If you have trouble, think of a style icon or a woman you admire. The goal here is for you to use this mental imagery to produce the positive picture of yourself you will then construct in reality using the tools in part II.

the most physical training. For years this study has encouraged people to combine imagination with execution in order to achieve the best results.

Famous celebrities have been known to employ this practice as well. My favorite example is the story of Jim Carrey, who wrote himself a check for $10 million in 1987 "for acting services rendered" and then carried it with him in his wallet throughout the ups and downs of his early acting career as a reminder of his ultimate goal. The check was dated Thanksgiving 1995, and in 1994 he earned $10 million for his film work. He has since stated that he visualized his future success and that this exercise helped him get there.

This theory can easily apply to your style as well. By combining your personality, character traits, and attributes, your likes, and the images and inspiration in your style file, you can start painting a mental picture of your ideal *you*. Since style is inherently creative and visual, it stands to reason that engaging in creative visualization is a good precursor to achieving your desired style.

LOVE VERSUS FEAR

Last, make sure you commit out of love, not fear. I've always felt that people approach life and all its challenges from one of two places: love or fear. Those working from love handle things with consideration, care, and purity, whereas those operating from fear can be driven by insecurity, ego, or a need for control. People who come from love include those friends who are selfless, who want you to succeed and will do whatever they can, even if it might be inconvenient for them to help you. They are the coworkers who are happy for you even when you're promoted over them, the significant others who are proud, not jealous, when you're hit on. Fear-based people function from self-doubt and can therefore end up doing things for the wrong reasons.

I want you to commit to your style out of love, because you know you deserve to feel strong and empowered every day and you want to take positive steps to improve your life and attract good things. Don't do this because you're afraid you won't get the job or the guy if you don't "change" or because you want to compete with anyone else. The best, most enriching, and longest-lasting results occur when, with pure intentions and strong self-confidence, we commit to making a lifestyle change.

Now that you understand that maintaining an accurate and self-fulfilling style is a process requiring commitment, you're ready to dive into part II. It's time to learn about all the style tools available to help you on this journey and how to amplify all the elements already working in your favor. Together, we will take everything you've discovered so far and use it to visually put *you* out into the universe.

> "At the moment of commitment the entire universe conspires to assist you."
>
> —JOHANN WOLFGANG VON GOETHE

And so do I.

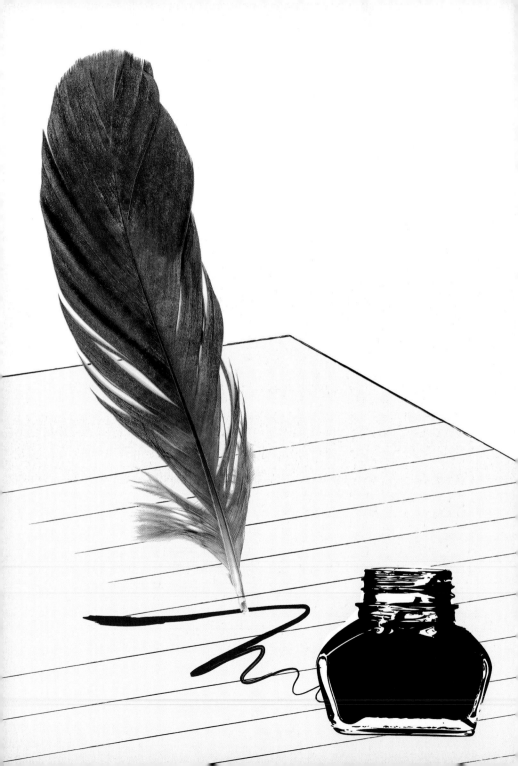

INTERLUDE

You've assembled all the tools needed to build your style; now it's time to put them to use. Your commitment is the bridge connecting your awareness to your execution, your inside to your outside. It's what will move you to action and ensure that the world sees the *you* you want them to see. To help make the jump easier, let's review all the observations you've accumulated, so you're ready, willing, and able to implement your style on a daily basis.

While reading the following pages, keep in mind all the notes you took throughout part I. Also keep in mind any would-you questions that apply to you and your life.

5 STEPS TO WEARING YOUR STYLE INSIDE OUT

1. SEE YOURSELF

Remember: *Work on manifesting a healthier image. Don't approach a mirror on a seek-and-destroy mission. Use the mirrors around you (your friends, your home, the way you carry yourself) to brilliantly reinforce and reflect your best qualities.*

2. ACT THE PART

Remember: *Body language is the only constant form of communication. Over 90 percent of communication is nonverbal, so be aware of what your body language, demeanor, and overall style are saying about you. Make sure your verbal and nonverbal messages are in sync. Pay attention to how people react to you when you first meet them and what they are reacting to. Use nonverbal communication to reinforce, not compete, with your personality, goals, and interests. Appearances matter.*

3. SPEAK UP

Remember: *Your style is a layer of language you wear, communicating on your behalf and being perceived by others. Consider yourself a brand worthy of accurate promotion, and understand who you are and what you want to say. Use your style speak to pinpoint your message based on your goals and intentions.*

4. KNOW YOUR WORTH

Remember: *Make sure you place your value in constant, intrinsic qualities that can't be taken away. Accept yourself and know that you're worth the time, energy, and effort it takes to invest in yourself and your packaging. And share your gifts with others.*

5. PUT A PLAN INTO PRACTICE

Remember: *You are your own priority, and input equals output, so put effort into committing to your own style journey. Set a style budget, find time for fittings, and conjure up an ideal version of you as your goal to achieve in part II.*

The fashion, accessory, and beauty choices you make should be consistent with your responses to these steps—with the way you see yourself and want to be seen by others. So allow your thoughts, feelings, likes, and dislikes to influence the style decisions you make moving forward. Use this reference whenever you need a reminder throughout part II to help you become your best, most stylish self.

PART II

BRINGING THE INSIDE OUT

Now it's time to wear yourself out . . . without wearing yourself out. (That's why I'm here.) Let's harness the power of your packaging.

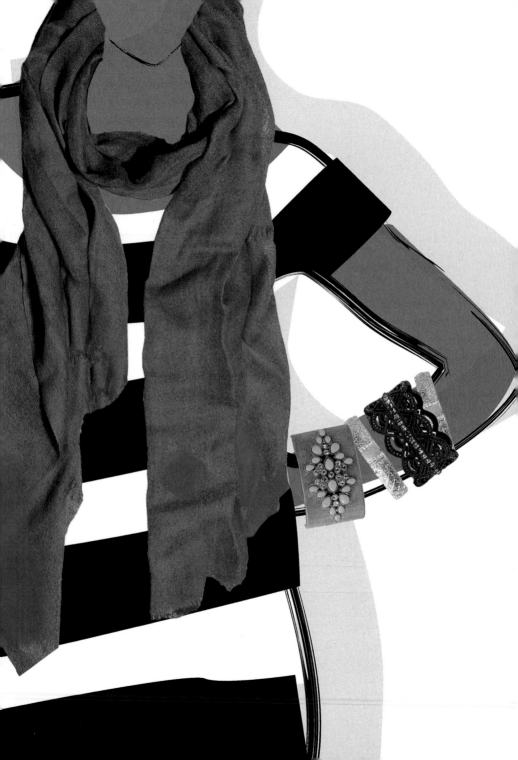

LEARN YOUR COLORS

Do you have a favorite color? If so, do you think you could explain why it's your favorite? Do you consciously surround yourself with blue because it makes you feel happy or calm? Maybe you feel powerful as a result of the compliments you get when you're wearing green? Many of us, whether we're aware of it or not, are instinctively drawn to hues that make us feel good in one way or another. Now that you have a clearer idea of all the parts of the inner you that you want to strengthen and express via your style, it's time to enhance things on the outside. One of the most powerful styling tools you have at your disposal, and the first place I like to start when talking about fashion, is color. It's something that surrounds you every day and is already hanging in your closet.

Not only do colors carry with them certain associations that can help you attract the things you want and make stronger style statements, but they can also visually alter your look in dramatic ways. Have you ever had one of those in-the-dumps days when you say to yourself "I look awful" or "I need more sleep"? You'd be surprised at how a simple color change can help you look more alert, improve your mood, and visually brighten you up. On the flip side, if you're wearing a color unsuited to your specific complexion, it has the potential to wash you out, highlight imperfections like dark circles or fine lines, or cause you to appear run-down. This is why it's so important to know which colors work best, not only for your physical makeup, such as your skin tone and features, but also for specific circumstances. When you use color to your advantage, to accentuate your features instead of compete with them, and to reinforce your messages, it will further articulate your style speak. Best of all, it's a great place to begin building a flattering wardrobe, since you can start with items you already own. So let's break it down to the basics: cool and warm colors.

TAKE THE TEMPERATURE: WARM VERSUS COOL

When you were a child someone probably taught you about the three primary colors: red, yellow, and blue. Little did you know that this was one lesson you could use throughout your life. These colors, often abbreviated as RYB, are important points on the color wheel, because all other hues on the spectrum are created from some mixture of these original three. While crayons and finger painting likely taught you that red and blue make purple, the process and combinations get much more specific from this point on. The generally accepted color wheel is composed of twelve basic hues formed by first mixing the primary colors to make green, orange, and violet,

then further mixing each of these secondary colors with the original RYB primary colors to create the tertiary colors: yellow-green,
yellow-orange, red-orange, red-violet, blue-violet, and blue-green.

Some of you might remember television sets from twenty or thirty
years ago and the minuscule RYB lights in the screens, which dis-
played moving colored images. Today, computers and software programs, like Photoshop and even Microsoft Word, allow you to run
your mouse over a color wheel to choose custom color combinations
of the primary three. Because of this continuous blending of colors
on the spectrum, it's possible to, as color experts would say, "take
the temperature of a color."

Though the RYB composition of every color is unique, all colors can be placed into one of two groups: warm or cool. These two
distinct categories divide a basic twelve-hue color wheel in half.
Hues from red through yellow, including browns, are considered
warm, while hues from blue-green through blue-violet, including
most grays, are considered cool, though potentially every hue has a
warmer or cooler version that isn't reflected on the basic wheel.

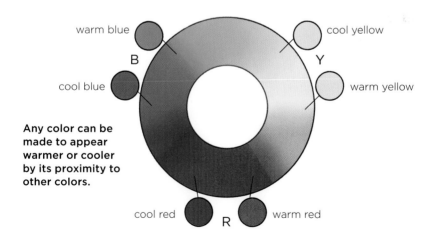

warm blue

cool blue

B

cool yellow

warm yellow

Y

**Any color can be
made to appear
warmer or cooler
by its proximity to
other colors.**

cool red

warm red

R

WARM IF BY LAND

To state the obvious, warm colors evoke feelings of warmth: fire, heat, etc. I like to take it a step further and call these the land colors. Think of rolling hills, lush harvests, golden sunsets, the vast landscapes of deserts, and rich red earth. These are your browns, orange-reds, dusty yellows, and earthy forest greens.

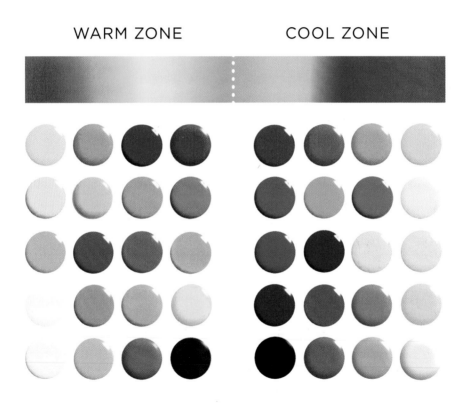

COOL IF BY SEA

Cool colors, on the other hand, are meant to conjure feelings of cold, ice, etc. I call these the sea colors. Whenever I envision the cool color palette, my mind immediately goes to deep ocean waters, the jewel tones associated with sunken treasures, and all the blues, emerald greens, and purples associated with this.

YOUR COLOR CATEGORY

We all came into this world with a unique physical and chemical makeup. Whether you have stayed au naturel over the years, experimented with various hair colors, laid out in the sun, or indulged in spray tans, try to think back to your original state. The first way to determine whether you're a warm or cool person—what we'll refer to from this point on as your coloring—is by assessing your skin tone and skin undertone. While they sound similar, these two are different and easy to confuse, so let me help set the record straight.

Your skin tone is essentially the color of your skin, regardless of whether it is fair, medium, or dark. There are hundreds of variations among all races and ethnicities. Since our society is comprised of a beautiful blend of people, and skin tones are far more nuanced than ever before, this can lead to mislabeling by anyone who still thinks coloring has everything to do with the color of your skin. It does not.

While your skin tone can help you gauge your best colors, your skin's undertone often plays the larger role. Undertone refers to whether you look better in warm or cool colors, and there are a few factors that influence this, regardless of your skin tone. Generally, the warm and cool categories are classified as follows:

Your Glow

WARM = SUNLIGHT
A golden, yellowish, or peach skin tone with green undertones.

COOL = MOONLIGHT
A beige, pink, or rosy skin tone with blue, purple undertones.

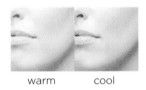
warm   cool

**FAIR
SKIN TONES**

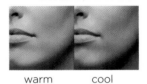
warm   cool

**MEDIUM
SKIN TONES**

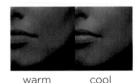
warm   cool

**DARK
SKIN TONES**

Plenty of factors make it difficult to immediately identify whether you are warm or cool, so try to make sure you are really looking for undertones. For example, if you have rosacea, don't automatically assume you are cool because of a pink tint; if you are of Asian or East Indian descent and have a yellowish pigment to your skin tone, you aren't necessarily warm; and if you are African American or have naturally dark skin that dominates your undertone, you may need to experiment with color swatches or look at pictures of yourself in order to find which category is most flattering for you. If you are still unclear about whether you are warm or cool, consider getting a professional color analysis.

Temperature Test

Are you warm or cool? These quick self-assessments can help you determine. (Beware of the yellow cast of incandescent light-bulbs. Perform these tests under natural lighting.)

1. Look at the inside of your wrists. Do your veins appear more bluish-purple or more green? If they appear blue, you are likely cool. If they seem green, you are probably warm. This is not a de-finitive test; some people either can't make out the color of their veins or may see both colors present. So let's go a step further.

2. Hold up a piece of crisp white paper next to your face. Do you notice more of a yellow-redness to your face (warm) or a blue-pink (cool)? Remember, you aren't looking directly at your skin, rather at the tone under your skin color reflecting against the page. If you're still not sure, maybe jewelry can help.

3. Do you tend to wear more silver or gold jewelry? Gold generally compliments warmer individuals while silver looks best on those who are cooler. If you're unsure, use jewelry, accessories, or clothing to note which of the two metallic tones flatters you. In a pinch, you can even try a sheet of aluminum foil as a stand-in for silver.

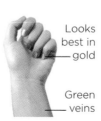

Looks best in gold

Looks best in silver

Green veins

Purple or blue veins

WARM

COOL

CONNECTING COLOR TO YOU

While fine-tuning your best colors is a rewarding process, it can be intimidating when you consider all the available research that has formed the systems used today. Philosophers and artists have been analyzing color for centuries. However, it wasn't until the 1940s that it became a popular practice to look at color from the perspective of clothing and style, when Suzanne Caygill, widely considered the pioneer of color analysis, developed what is now known as the Caygill Method of Seasonal Color Analysis. Then in 1980 Carole Jackson's *Color Me Beautiful* book, inspired by Caygill's method, became a pop-culture phenomenon. Jackson's system, although popular and easy to understand, was criticized because its inherent simplicity didn't account for variations in darker skin tones. Jackson acknowledged that it wasn't a perfect system and, as a result, dominant color analysis emerged, which focuses on a person's dominant features and characteristics rather than solely on skin tone. So, when it comes to breaking down your unique coloring and deciding which category best fits you, there is plenty of research available to help you delve as far into color as you'd like.

At the very least, simply knowing whether you are warm or cool is tremendously helpful. Yet it can be beneficial to also identify either a season or a dominant category to further narrow the field of colors best for you. To help you with this, take a look at the seasonal and dominant color analysis on pages 124 through 131.

Ideally, after looking at these charts you will have connected with a category based on your current coloring. But if this is challenging for you, a color correction may be needed. If you have al-tered your hair color or your skin tone has changed over the years (perhaps as a result of sun exposure), you might be inspired to go back to your roots and embrace your natural skin tone by slathering on the SPF and staying away from the self-bronzer. Or perhaps the opposite is true for you and some self-tanner and highlights could help you more closely align with one of the categories. The world is a mixing bowl with an unlimited blend of unique people, and some of you may overlap between seasons or dominant categories. It's up to you to alter, adjust, or borrow your best colors.

The general goal behind the color categories presented is to help you form a mental picture of which colors are naturally more flattering for you. But to personalize your palette, I'd like you to create your own color compass, one that takes into account your unique personality, likes and dislikes, and simplifies the colors, while still giving you direction and freedom to control what works for you.

YOUR COLOR COMPASS

From researching articles and TV segments to teaching color classes in malls across the country, I've had thousands of faces come up to me and ask me to instantly assess "Am I warm?" "Am I cool?" "Can I wear yellow? Pink?" Encountering hair from fire-engine-dyed red to blue-gray and every color skin tone in between, I was inspired to create a quick reference to help accurately guide you toward your best colors. I call this your custom color compass (see page 133 for an example).

SEASONAL COLOR ANALYSIS

WARM SEASONS

AUTUMN

Autumns are part of the warm category, with green undertones, and often have low-contrast features. Not all but a majority of people with

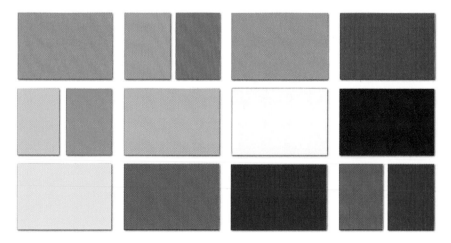

AUTUMNS: Have warm coloring and low contrast

brown hair and brown eyes fall into this category, as do most classic red-heads. They may appear to have an overall rich, spicy coloring. If you are an autumn, you look best in earthy as well as muted warm colors, such as spicy reds, burnt oranges, moss greens, and deep plums. Your best neutrals would be cream and dark chocolate brown.

Autumns: Susan Sarandon, Beyoncé, Julia Roberts, Eva Mendes

SPRING

Springs are also part of the "warm" complexion category, with green undertones, and they tend to have low-contrasting features. Many springs have an overall clear, golden coloring and look best wearing golden browns, corals, peaches, yellow greens, and aquas. For neutrals, go with ivory instead of white and golden brown instead of black.

Springs: Jennifer Aniston, Nicole Kidman, Reba McEntire, Rashida Jones

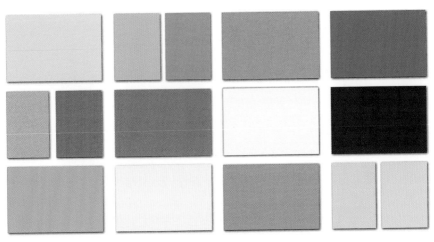

SPRINGS: Tend to have warm coloring and low contrast

COOL SEASONS

WINTER

Winters are classified as those cool people with blue skin undertones, who usually possess a high contrast between their hair, skin, and eye color. This typically means they have darker hair and lighter skin and eyes. Their coloring can be referred to as crisp and distinctive, and they look best in similar bright, deep colors, such as navy, emerald green, hot pink, and true red. As far as neutrals, winters should wear stark, crisp white and clear black.

Winters: Elizabeth Taylor, Courtney Cox, Brooke Shields, Anne Hathaway, Ann Curry

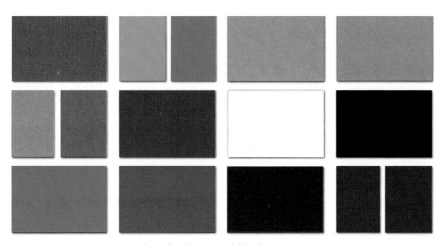

WINTERS: Have cool coloring and high contrast

SUMMER

Summers also fall under the cool category but generally have a low contrast between their hair, skin, and eye color, meaning everything is similar in intensity (e.g., light eyes paired with light hair). Summers may be referred to as having a "soft and subtle" appearance and seem to have a more neutral (sometimes beige in lighter skin tones) coloring. They can lean toward presenting an overall ashy tone rather than a golden one. If you are a summer, you look best in cool, muted colors, including most blues (blue-gray, periwinkle, etc.), lavender, pastel pinks, and browns. When it comes to neutrals, opt for sand or soft white and slate gray or charcoal.

Summers: Farrah Fawcett, Rihanna, Jodie Foster

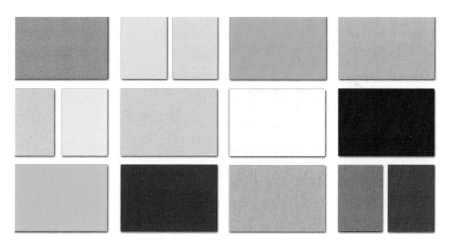

SUMMERS: Have cool coloring and low contrast

DOMINANT COLOR ANALYSIS

Often people have a difficult time fitting into a specific season. If you don't feel you fit neatly into one season over the others, dominant characteristic color analysis might work better for you. Try to discern your most striking characteristic, and then take a look at the following dominant color chart to see which category suits you. The dominant system focuses more on whether you are deep, light, soft, clear, warm, or cool rather than relying so heavily on your skin undertones.

Deep

Characteristics: Deep features that are bold, dramatic, and dominate (dark hair, dark eyes). Although your skin tone may be fair, many African American and Hispanic people fit into this category.

Deep Warms include: Julia Roberts, Eva Mendes, Jennifer Lopez, Keira Knightley, Penelope Cruz, Freida Pinto, Oprah Winfrey, Margaret Cho. This category is also sometimes known as Deep Autumn.

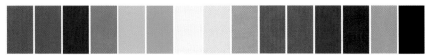

Deep Cools include: Sandra Bullock, Anne Hathaway, Victoria Beckham, Demi Moore, Lucy Liu, Kim Kardashian. This category is also sometimes known as Deep Winter.

Light

Characteristics: Light, delicate coloring overall. Generally light eyes, light hair, and fair skin that lack contrast.

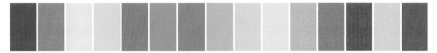

Light Warms include: Taylor Swift, Ellen DeGeneres, Blake Lively, Anna Kournikova. This category is also sometimes known as Light Spring.

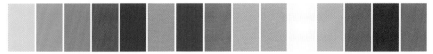

Light Cools include: Reese Witherspoon, Scarlett Johansson, Diane Sawyer, Naomi Watts, Gwyneth Paltrow. This category is also sometimes known as Light Summer.

Soft

Characteristics: Soft, neutral, muted features. A blend of both warm and cool characteristics. Multiracial people, or those with lighter shades of the dark skin tones who have light eyes, often fall into this group.

Soft Warms include: Jennifer Aniston, Gisele Bündchen, Rihanna, Jada Pinkett Smith, Drew Barrymore. This category is also sometimes known as Soft Autumn.

Soft Cools include: Sarah Jessica Parker, Annette Bening. This category is also sometimes known as Soft Summer.

Clear

Characteristics: Overall clear coloring that is vivid and crisp. There is often a high contrast between hair, skin, and eyes (e.g., dark hair with bright eyes).

Clear Warms include: Katie Holmes, Elizabeth Hurley, Sophia Bush, Adriana Lima. This category is also sometimes known as Clear Spring.

Clear Cools include: Courtney Cox, Megan Fox, Liv Tyler. This category is also sometimes known as Clear Winter.

Warm

Characteristics: Warm, golden features overall. This group includes nearly all classic redheads.

Warm Lights include: Amy Adams, Shirley MacLaine, Nicole Kidman. This category is also sometimes known as Warm Spring.

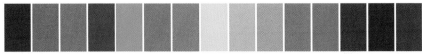

Warm Mediums include: Debra Messing, Sophia Loren, Beyoncé, Halle Berry. This category is also sometimes known as Warm Autumn.

Cool

Characteristics: Cool features overall with ashy, blue, or pink undertones.

Cool Mediums include: Kate Middleton, Miranda Lambert, Paulina Porizkova, Judi Dench. This category is also sometimes known as Cool Summer.

Cool Darks include: Elizabeth Taylor, Brooke Shields, Jennifer Connelly. This category is also sometimes known as Cool Winter.

Based on whether you identify as a warm- or cool-colored person, I want you to fill in this chart with the answers to the questions that follow it.

Light: _____

Dark: _____

Neutral: _____

Power: _____

Favorite: _____

Seasonals (Fall and Summer): _____

What's your best light color: white or ivory?

What's your best dark color: black or chocolate brown?

What's your best neutral color: beige, gray, or camel?

What's your power color, your most complimentary color based on your color analysis—the color that pops up in both the seasonal and the dominant analysis?

What's your favorite color, the color you like best—probably what you own the most of? It could be but doesn't have to be included in your color analysis.

What are your seasonal colors, the two colors you most easily incorporate during the cool months (winter and fall) and the warm months (spring and summer) and that usually align with your color analysis?

To help guide you, I'm including my own color compass (as an example of cool) as well as my friend Maggie's (an example of warm).

Bobbie's Color Compass

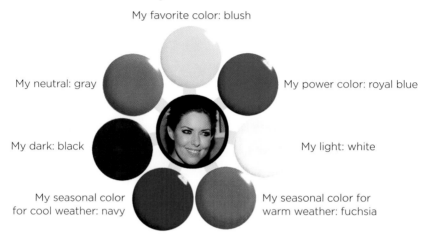

My favorite color: blush

My neutral: gray

My power color: royal blue

My dark: black

My light: white

My seasonal color for cool weather: navy

My seasonal color for warm weather: fuchsia

Maggie's Color Compass

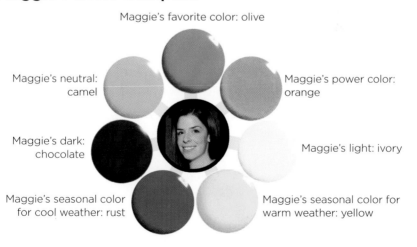

Maggie's favorite color: olive

Maggie's neutral: camel

Maggie's power color: orange

Maggie's dark: chocolate

Maggie's light: ivory

Maggie's seasonal color for cool weather: rust

Maggie's seasonal color for warm weather: yellow

The goal here is to help simplify your style process by isolating your best and favorite colors. I want you to create a snapshot of the seven colors (including both seasonals, fall and summer) to keep in mind or even carry with you on a small card tucked in your wallet to reference when you're shopping. The idea behind both the seasonal color analysis and my custom color compass is to find out what works for you. As Coco Chanel said, "The best color in the whole world is the one that looks good on you." Who wouldn't want to have a secret weapon of a specific color to stand out in a crowd?

This information is intended to help you cut the clutter. There are limitless hues to choose from in the spectrum, but in reality, when you have the basic understanding of what works for you, you can build a wardrobe around these key colors, accenting as you see fit. It's to help you keep in mind the most flattering direction for you, plus get you more bang for your buck. When you invest in colors that flatter you, you'll

> **"The best color in the whole world is the one that looks good on you."**
>
> **—Coco Chanel**

be more inclined to wear those items, since you'll have confidence in your choices. Sticking with your personal seven best colors can help you build a wardrobe that is interchangeable and works well together.

WEAR THE "WRONG" COLOR RIGHT

Circumstances will pop up when you either want to or have to wear a color that doesn't fall into your category (e.g., you have to wear a bridesmaid's dress or a uniform). You will likely fall in love with a dress, skirt, or sweater from time to time that isn't in your seven colors or even in your season. Maybe you'll really want to jump into a current color trend (like neon), even though you know it doesn't mesh with your coloring. This is okay! You can wear any color you want to because, first, you are your own person and entitled to express yourself however you see fit and, second, no one is going to physically stop you. Having said that, a few tricks of the trade will ensure you still flatter your unique features and help you wear the "wrong" color right.

Styling Tips

Scarves and Statement Necklaces: A simple scarf in one of your complimentary colors can be your best friend. I almost never leave home without one. It can save you from the sun and warm you from a chill, but beyond that, whether you drape it across your shoulders or twist it into a temporary necklace, it frames your face. A statement necklace in a flattering hue works the same way. Both items draw the eye upward, allowing you to wear any color you wish below.

Patterns: If you love a certain shade that doesn't work for you, look for it in a print that includes a complimentary color. Many designers are aware that not every hue looks good on every person, so they combine colors from opposite sides of the spectrum. This way the color you love can still be the focal point of your ensemble, but you can use your accessories (belt, shoes, handbag) to bring out your more flattering color from within the pattern.

Beauty Tricks

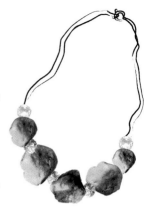

Body: You can add warmth, if you fall under the cool category, by trying a body shimmer in gold. This tricks the eye into making your skin undertone appear warmer, allowing you to wear a warmer-colored garment. To achieve the reverse, apply a body shimmer with a silver base.

Blush: If you are warm, your undertone may have a peach hue to it. Counteract this with a pink-peach blush to give your face a slightly cooler tone. Then you are better able to wear cooler colors around your face. If you are cool and looking to wear a warm color, the opposite will work for you and you should wear a peach-based blush.

Lips: Like blush, add a pop of lip color that includes a subtle shade of an opposite hue. If you are cool, a beige or blush lip color with hints of peach or coral can help you wear warm colors. If you are on the warmer side, move away from an orangey rust and try a deep brown or red that's more neutral.

Eye Shadow: For warm gals looking to wear cool dresses, warm up your face with a smoky brown eye shadow to pull the attention up from a gray or navy dress. For cools, go with a gray or blue eye shadow to take the focus off a brown or similarly warm ensemble.

Nails: Pull a flattering background color from a print or enhance your own coloring with the exclamation point of a nail polish in a complimentary color.

THE PSYCHOLOGY OF COLOR

As I mentioned in the beginning of this step, it's equally important to understand not only what colors best flatter your features but also the psychology behind your color choices. You now know that your style speak sends a loud message, and color can either strengthen or distract from what you are communicating. Think about if you've ever gone to a party where most everyone was wearing some variation of a little black dress. (This has happened to me.) Wouldn't you respond to the one woman wearing bold yellow? Of course you would, and so would everyone else. What you have to keep in mind is the situation. If this were a birthday or cocktail party with friends, wearing a well-chosen yellow instead of a safe black choice would probably garner positive attention and compliments, whereas if the occasion were an after-work happy hour, the color could come across as overpowering.

Knowing your seven colors helps to ensure that you're visually sending your best self out into the universe. Yet your efforts can be undone if you don't connect the color to the context.

Color and Common Sense

When choosing a color, consider the context and what you're trying to say. Since all colors carry with them certain associations, be they cultural, historical, or emotional, you want to be sure your intentions are not being misinterpreted.

Much like you would take into account your setting, when assessing how comfortable you are with what you're wearing, also consider your color choice, since each hue carries with it a connota-

Color Your Word

In step 3, "Speak Up," we discussed three worthwhile adjectives to keep in mind, taking into account your daily goals when deciding what to wear. Here, I would like you to think of what colors you can pair with your adjectives to further strengthen your style speak. I have included my adjectives and corresponding colors to help guide you.

STRIKING . . . When I want to stand out or be memorable, I usually look to my power color as a base. For me, this is royal or electric blue.

CHIC . . . When the goal is to be graceful and stylish without being flashy, I often look to my light and dark colors as my base. These are white and black for me. (I say "base" because when I've built my wardrobe around these base colors, it's easier to add accessories or accents in other colors depending on how I feel.)

INVITING . . . When I aim to be welcoming, I often turn to either my neutral or my favorite color as a base. For me, gray and beige are the ones I tend to feel the most relaxed in.

tion that resonates with others. You want to be sure the take-away from your color choice is positive and powerful instead of distracting. Keep in mind that it's still somewhat subjective, and your body language and demeanor will go a long way to supporting your style speak, regardless of what color you're wearing. But color is a conscious decision and can leave a strong impression after you have left a room. While this may seem like yet another layer to consider, your newfound awareness of color will soon make the decision instinctual and become part of your routine.

COLOR AND STYLE SPEAK

Experts in the fields of art, fashion, and design have studied the meanings and implications of color for years. However, when color is put into practical everyday use, few of us are realistically going to remember that green represents new beginnings before we get dressed for a baby shower. What you *will* remember is when your cousin's girlfriend wears electric pink to your great-grandmother's funeral. So while you absolutely want to express yourself and use color to reinforce your style speak, keep in mind that colors can say many different things.

 RED ───────────────────────────────

Red can be seen as romantic when worn on a dinner date or fun when you're out with friends. It can come off as powerful paired with a work suit or passionate and playful when worn in "pops."

Red can also come across as overpowering or aggressive if worn to an intimate event. If you're wearing a notice-me-now red to a formal or professional setting, it can appear overdone.

YELLOW

Yellow's inherent sunny associations can brighten up a room and send out positive, cheerful, and energetic messages. Fun and playful, the woman wearing yellow is likely someone you'll feel comfortable talking to.

Yellow can be distracting when the overall tone of a situation is somber or requires focus.

BLUE

Blue is often considered a calming color associated with trust and serenity. With so many variations, it's easy to wear almost anywhere.

Because of its versatility, blue can seem like a safe choice or even come across as boring if your goal is to wow.

GREEN

A down-to-earth color, green implies level-headedness and approachability.

Due to its link to nature, organics, and the outdoors, green can skew as more casual than some of the other colors, making it harder to dress up.

PURPLE

Very rarely found in nature, you almost have to go out of your way to wear purple. This effort evokes a sense of creativity, imagination, and fun.

With ties to imagination, purple is abundant in children's apparel, games, and toys and can therefore appear youthful.

ORANGE

The most energetic color, orange can send a bold style statement. Bright and warm, it's a color that attracts others and can come across as friendly and outgoing.

It can also come off as attention seeking, if worn out of context. Depending on how light or dark it is, it can give off a very season-specific vibe.

 ## BROWN

Brown is subtle but often less expected than black, and therefore it can be engaging. It's a practical color that conveys reliability.

Brown can appear dull or make the wearer seem disinterested if the context is fun or lively. It currently has a retro association that can come off as dated.

 ## GRAY

Gray is interestingly the easiest color for the eye to see and can evoke feelings of sophistication and intellect.

As a result of its associations with sadness and depression (e.g., gray days of winter) it's not typically a wise choice if you're looking to come across as spontaneous.

WHITE

The color most associated with purity, innocence, and cleanliness, white can help you look organized, responsible, and under control.

A color with many false rules associated with it (don't wear after Labor Day, before Memorial Day, to a wedding, etc.), white can help you stand out, so make sure that's part of your goal.

● BLACK ─────────────────────────────────

Black is considered a very powerful color and is often associated with elegance and chic.

Because of its prevalence, it can sometimes be seen as unimaginative or serious.

By no means is this chart an in-depth breakdown representative of each hue, but rather food for thought about the hues in general. Here are a few more broad strokes about color.

Neutrals: Neutrals are just that—they play well with others. They can come across as sophisticated, yet they are colors everyone wears, regardless of age. Both modern and mature, some people rely on them solely, while others pass them by in favor of bolder, more prominent hues. If you fall into the former category, just be sure you aren't using neutrals as a crutch or a safety blanket to cover up your true personality. On the other hand, if you hardly incorporate neutrals at all, these underrated colors can make great investment pieces and have a place of importance.

Brights: Inherent in the name, these are bold and powerful colors that should be worn when you want to be seen. I consider these scene-stealers, especially when worn in your most flattering colors. Be cautious of a hue that contrasts with your coloring, as it can over-power you or cause you to get lost.

Darks: Darks have a different kind of power. These are the more serious tones that are often viewed as responsible and trustworthy. Think back to black. This color can be seen as a boundary (a reason that many authority figures dress in black). However, you can also appear to be hiding behind it, shrouding yourself and telling the world to keep out. It can be a go-to color for people uncomfortable with their body image, a way to keep attention away.

Pastels: These light colors can come across as youthful, almost childlike, but when worn with sleek basics or a sophisticated neutral, they can offer refreshing twists. For example, when paired with black they can offer a modern edge; taupe or gray can age them up, making them more appropriate; and when worn with white, the effect can be eye-catching. Look to your color compass to best balance how to wear the hues you like the most.

Color is simply one more tool in your style kit to help you say what you want and, ultimately, get what you want. Connecting to your best colors can offer you an advantage, but in general, this step was meant to be colorful insight. I hope you break the rules and make exceptions to customize this color information. After all, confidence is still going to trump any small gain from choosing a blue over a green in a given circumstance.

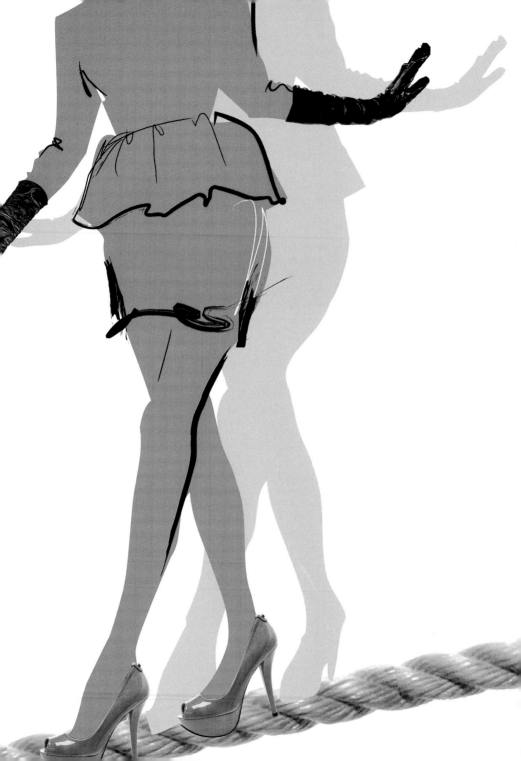

BALANCE YOUR BODY

If you've ever loved a dress on a friend and borrowed it only to realize it didn't look quite right on you, or been drawn to a trend, like high-waisted denim, but have never been able to find a pair that flatters, don't worry. You're not alone. Sadly, clothes aren't cut with every body in mind. While you can recite your jeans, dress, shirt, and shoe sizes off the top of your head, could you tell me what your body shape is? Have you ever

> **It's not about size; it's about shape.**

thought about it? If so, do you know what items work for or against your figure? We live in a three-dimensional world, so our challenge is finding the right fit from clothing that appears two-dimensional on a hanger. It's not about size; it's about shape.

Many people confuse body shape with size, but these two concepts couldn't be farther apart. Think about the common small, medium, and large charts many retailers use to help shoppers find their size. Have you ever stopped to realize that these charts are used to guide literally *everyone* into one of these preset groups? Occasionally certain stores offer an XS, XL, or XXL option, but in general, you, me, and everyone we know are all supposed to fit into one of six sizes. Similarly, not all size-12 women are the same height and weight, are they? To some extent, the number on the tag and the weight on the scale are arbitrary, since all clothing is going to fit different people differently.

The only way to ensure you choose clothes that best fit and flatter your unique body is to understand your general shape. You only get one body, so whether you're tall, short, curvy, slim, athletic, or your own unique mixture of them all, there are many basic tips, tricks, and guidelines to help you make informed choices when it comes to cuts and silhouettes.

BALANCE AND PROPORTION

Humans crave harmony, and whether you're a supermom or a supermodel, everyone's goal is visual balance. In fact, in a study conducted by Brunel University in the UK researchers created detailed virtual models of the bodies of seventy-seven adult human subjects and measured them for degrees of symmetry. To eliminate bias based on facial features or skin color, the heads of the virtual models were eliminated and the skin tones were all made the same neutral shade. The researchers then asked volunteers to rate the attractiveness of the opposite-sex models. Although the differences in symmetry were barely noticeable to the naked eye, both men and women reported that the symmetrical bodies were more attractive.

So, whether we are aware of it or not, we are naturally attracted to symmetry, and even the smallest changes can make a big difference.

Unfortunately, when it comes to our bodies, very, very, very few people are naturally symmetrical. But we can create this illusion with what we choose to wear. Whether you are a size 2 or 22, the goal is to balance your body using silhouettes, accents, and strategic color combinations best suited for you.

THE X FACTOR: KNOW YOUR BODY TYPE

You've had years to get familiar with your body, but if you're like most women, you probably still go through sessions of wardrobe trial and error, whether it's combining separates from your own closet, trying new trends, or moving outside your comfort zone. As an individual, I've gone through this with my own clothes over the years and had to figure out what looks best on my body. As a style editor, I've also had to become intimately and instantly familiar with complete strangers of all shapes and sizes, who depend on me to come up with the perfect outfit on the spot.

Born of necessity, the X factor appeared. I visually spot an X on someone's frame to quickly assess that person's body type, how I might balance his or her look, and in turn suggest the most flattering option. Seeing this mental mark allows me to envision an axis point from which to focus, as well as areas that should be highlighted or adjusted. The X factor can help you shift your mind to shift your shape. For every perceived problem area there is an equal and opposite positive area. Understanding this concept will spare you hours of frustration

> **Shift your mind to shift your shape.**

in front of your closet, save you decades of dressing-room drama, and give you hints when looking at something on the hanger.

We are all of various heights, we all carry weight a little differently, and all our body parts are uniquely our own. Yet most people typically identify with one of five general body types: hourglass, triangle, inverted triangle, diamond, or rectangle. To figure out which body type you fall under, all you have to do is find your X.

BODY TYPES

The body type you identify for yourself using the X factor is based on your skeletal frame. Therefore, certain details, including height, bust size, and weight, can and will vary on all individuals and across each of the five typical body types. This variation is what makes us all both common and unique; each group shares distinct attributes, yet a range of subtypes is possible within each. While you will typically remain the same body type, physical changes—such as pregnancy, significant weight loss or gain, aging—could cause your shape to shift from one type to another. Similarly, it's not uncommon to identify with more than one body type. Like your best colors, the five basic types are here to guide you. So if you find that some of your features are a combination of two different categories, that's fine. Feel free to borrow from both. Just keep in mind the reasoning behind why certain cuts fit and flatter your X factor better than others, and make your own rules.

ILLUSION = Proportion Play + Clever Use of Cut and Color

THE X FACTOR

ARE YOUR SHOULDERS AND HIPS EVEN?

And your waistline is defined? Then you're an hourglass.

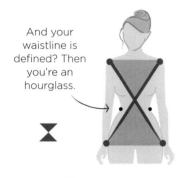

If your waist is in line with your shoulders and hips, you're a rectangle.

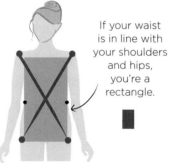

Is your waistline your widest point? Then you're a diamond.

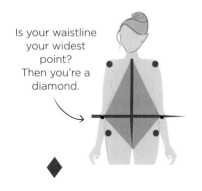

ARE YOUR SHOULDERS AND HIPS UNEVEN?

If your shoulders are narrower than your hips, you're a triangle.

If your hips are narrower than your shoulders, you're an inverted triangle.

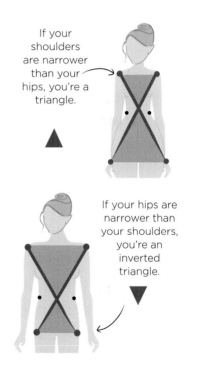

Still not sure of your shape? See style session "Find Your X" on page 150.

Find Your X

Grab a buddy, such as a friend or family member, because this style session requires the help of someone close. Stand with good posture and your arms relaxed at your sides in front of an all-white or solid-colored wall. You can wear a snug black outfit, or if you're up for it, a bathing suit or bra and underwear. Now have your style-session buddy snap a photo of you. The goal is to take a photo that will clearly capture the outline of your frame. Print it out and, using a pencil, mark the outermost points of your shoulders and hips. Then draw an X by connecting the dots. Next, note your waistline with dots, at the point underneath your ribcage and just above your belly button. If your waistline points measure wider than your hips and shoulders, your X will more closely resemble a cross. Just remember to be honest and accurate, and if you decided to strike a pose in the buff, be sure to delete the picture!

Hourglass   Triangle   Inverted Triangle   Rectangle   Diamond

REALITY CHECK

It's important to note that we all get stuck in ruts. It's impossible to be perfect, and there will definitely be those days when, no matter

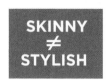

how great your intentions, you can't seem to get out of a funk. It's at times like these that knowing your body type and your most flattering silhouettes helps you work on what you can't see by focusing on what you can, even if it means you have to physically drag yourself out of bed, make yourself up, spritz on your favorite perfume, and wrap yourself in your most flattering cuts and colors. People say that when you feel good, you look good. While the exact opposite has also become somewhat of a cliché, I say that when you look good, you at least feel better. Life doesn't have to start five pounds from now and it didn't end

> **Work on what you can't see by focusing on what you can.**

five years ago. So allow this information about body shapes to build you up and ensure that you are using fashion as a way to reflect the best version of who you are today and every day.

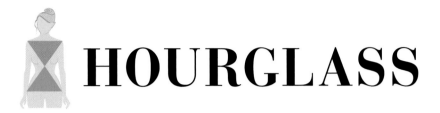# HOURGLASS

If your X intersects in the middle of your body, you likely have an hourglass figure. Those of you blessed with this balanced shape naturally align, meaning the width of your shoulders and hips are proportional.

BODY BLOCKING

Dark Areas: Diminish with deeper colors, neutrals, solids, and vertical lines.

Light Areas: Draw attention to with bright colors, prints, texture, and horizontal lines.

The hourglass shape is naturally balanced. You can maintain your symmetry by highlighting your midsection. Unlike the other body types, who can use body blocking to adjust their X factors, your goal is to avoid imbalance. As an hourglass, you want to showcase your waist and let your natural curves speak for themselves. Therefore, the shading in this illustration is the reverse of the other body types. I realize (as an hourglass myself) you may want to elongate your

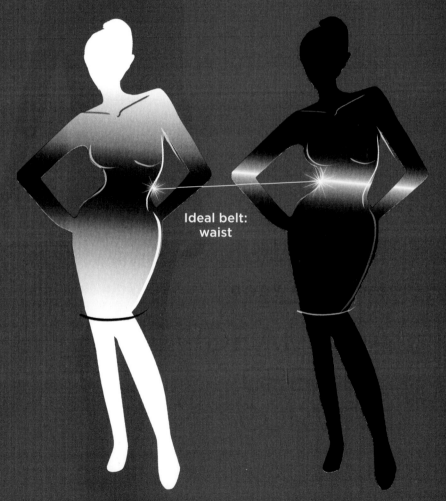

BODY BLOCKING

IDEAL GOAL: CONTROL YOUR CURVES

Ideal belt:
waist

PLAY 'EM UP   —OR—   PLAY 'EM DOWN

frame. This requires minimizing your curves and, in turn,
creates more of a rectangle
effect, employing the opposite
shading principals the other
types use for body blocking.

> **"Your dresses should be tight enough to know you're a woman, and loose enough to show you're a lady."**
>
> **—Edith Head**

DRESSES

Curve Control: Highlight your waist and always consider your mid-section a focal point. Emphasize your proportionate figure, rather than allowing it to get lost in loose or baggy silhouettes.

Look For:

Leave Behind:

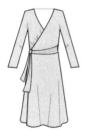 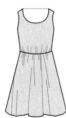 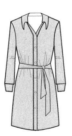 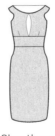 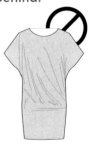

Wrap designs	Fit-and-flare styles	Belted options	Sheath and tailored cuts	Drop-waist and shapeless shifts, which create a boxy look

TOPS

"Girlfriends": If you're gifted up top, avoid loose blouses that billow or flare from the bustline, as they can add unnecessary volume.

Look For:

Leave Behind:

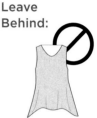

Tailored shirts and blazers	Form-fitted tops with darts	Cinched, banded, or belted blouses	V-necks and open necklines	Trapeze tops, which add bulk

BOTTOMS

Keep It Classy: Avoid shorter hemlines (miniskirts, "booty" shorts, etc.) unless you're petite (under five feet two inches tall). Your voluptuous figure offers enough sex appeal.

Look For:

Leave Behind:

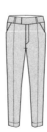
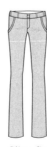

Pencil skirts	Tulip styles	Cropped trousers	Slim-fit bootleg cuts	Gathered waist or pleated styles, which add volume

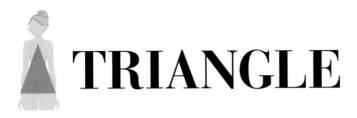

TRIANGLE

If your shoulders are narrower in proportion to your hips, with your X intersecting above your waist, you likely have a triangle body type.

BODY BLOCKING ➤

Dark Areas: Diminish with deeper colors, neutrals, solids, and vertical lines.

Light Areas: Draw attention to with bright colors, prints, texture, and horizontal lines.

As a triangle, you can balance your X factor by pulling the focus up to your shoulders and neckline. Wear visual interest—such as vibrant shades, lighter hues, and high-contrast patterns that demand attention—high (above your natural waistline), to transfer some of the power from the bottom of your X to the upper half. You can easily take advantage of trends like bold shoulders and statement necklaces or have fun with detailed tops.

IDEAL GOAL:
PLAY UP
THE TOP

Ideal belt:
empire waist

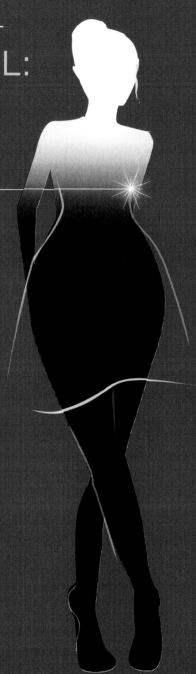

DRESSES

BFF Buys: Flirty frocks are your best friends, thanks to design elements that will flatter your frame.

Look For:

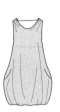 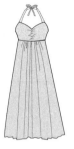 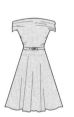 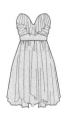

Leave Behind:

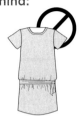

| Flowing trapeze styles | Halter necks and empire waistlines | Off-the-shoulder and fit-and-flare designs | Strapless styles and frills on top | Drop-waist dresses, which draw attention to the widest point of your body and conceal your natural waistline |

TOPS

Notice-Me Necklines: To best accentuate your X and balance your lower half, look for styles that draw attention to your delicate top half. Embrace embellishments or ruffles; flutter, princess, or puff sleeves; and more.

Look For:

Leave Behind:

| Boat- or wide-neck styles | Tops with built-in volume | Shoulder details and tie-neck blouses | Details at bust or neckline | Batwing and dolman sleeve tops, which hide your waistline and add bulk to your frame |

BOTTOMS

Hip, Hip, Hooray: Be confident that your curves are your hippest asset! Own your shape and show it off with skirts and dresses that skim your body and pants with clean lines and simple stitching.

Look For:

Leave Behind:

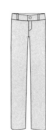

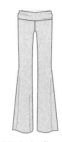

Knee-length A-line skirts

Full, high-waisted skirts

Flat-front, bootcut pants

Slightly flared yoga and palazzo pants

Voluminous bubble and pleated skirts, which add excess to your lower, dominant half

> **"Clothes are but a symbol of something hid deep beneath."**
>
> **—Virginia Woolf**

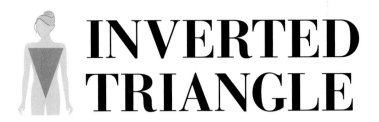

INVERTED TRIANGLE

When your hips are narrower in proportion to your shoulders, and your X intersects below your waist, you have an inverted-triangle silhouette.

BODY BLOCKING

Dark Areas: Diminish with deeper colors, neutrals, solids, and vertical lines.

Light Areas: Draw attention to with bright colors, prints, texture, and horizontal lines.

As an inverted triangle, the upper half of your X dominates the lower, so you want to draw the focus down to your hips to shift some of the power. Shorter-length skirts and dresses, lighter denim hues, fun patterned pants, and colorful shorts will help highlight your legs. And be sure to have fun with your footwear. Ankle straps, booties, and other statement shoes will add balance to your shoulders.

Ideal belt: hips

BODY BLOCKING

IDEAL GOAL: PLAY UP THE BOTTOM

> "It's not really a shorter skirt.
> I just have longer legs."
>
> —Anna Kournikova

DRESSES

You've Got Legs: And now you'll know how to use them! When it comes to dresses, look for those that are minimal and clean up top. Balance your hips and shoulders with full-skirted dresses, or show off how easily you can don a drop waist.

Look For:

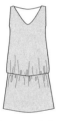

Drop-waist
styles

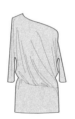

Draped,
loose
dresses

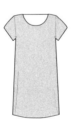

Shorter
shapeless
shifts

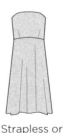

Strapless or
collarless
dresses

**Leave
Behind:**

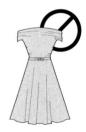

Off-the-shoulder
necklines and fit-
and-flare styles,
which highlight
your widest point
and box up your
frame

TOPS

Drop Tops: Opt for styles that hug you below your natural waistline or draw attention down with prints, trimming, etc.

Look For:

Leave Behind:

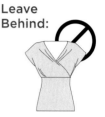

| Raglan sleeve tops | V-necks and tunics | Trapeze-style tops | Batwing and dolman sleeves | Tops with built-in volume, which visually bulk up shoulders or bust |

BOTTOMS

Sleek and Chic: Streamline your lower half and show off your legs.

Look For:

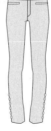

Leave Behind:

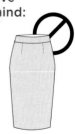

Shorter skirts

Pleated, ruffled, or flouncy skirts

Relaxed shorts

Slim-leg pants and leggings

Longer pencil skirts, which exaggerate the difference between your top and bottom halves

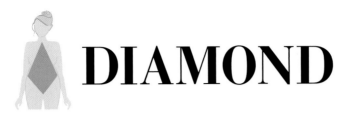

DIAMOND

If your hips and shoulders are proportionate, with your waist being the widest part of your frame, and your X appears tilted on its axis, you have a diamond silhouette.

BODY BLOCKING

Dark Areas: Diminish with deeper colors, neutrals, solids, and vertical lines.

Light Areas: Draw attention to with bright colors, prints, texture, and horizontal lines.

As a diamond, balance your body by shifting the focus inward. Light, bright shades and bold prints call attention, so wear these in vertical panels to elongate your frame. Look for detailing and patterns that move the eye up and down. Necklines and cuts that accentuate your shoulders and bust will work well for you. Show off your arms and legs, and take advantage of long, draping statement necklaces and slim scarves.

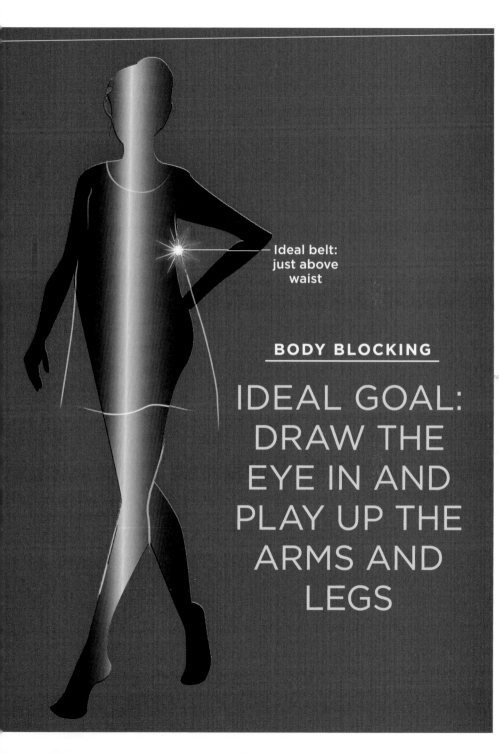

Ideal belt:
just above
waist

BODY BLOCKING

IDEAL GOAL: DRAW THE EYE IN AND PLAY UP THE ARMS AND LEGS

DRESSES

Line It Up: Vertical seams, zippers, pleating, and contrast stitching will visually stretch your frame.

Look For:

Leave Behind:

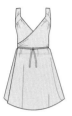
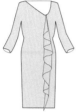
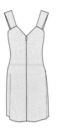
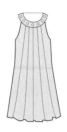
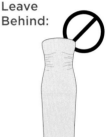

| Dresses lightly belted above the waist | Vertical details that elongate | Y-shaped dresses | Halter necklines | Tube-type dresses, which are unforgiving and emphasize horizontal proportions |

TOPS

Versatile V-Necks: From casual tees and classic tunics to sexy deeper cuts, they will frame your face and flatter your figure.

Look For:

Leave Behind:

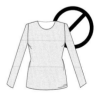

| Halters and front-twist designs | Boat and scoop necks | Playful sleeves and bustlines | V-neck tunics | Clingy, tight tops, which reveal any extra around the midriff |

BOTTOMS

Straight and Narrow: Not too wide nor too tapered, but just right. Look for bottoms that lengthen your lower half.

Look For:

Leave Behind: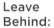

High-waisted sleek skirts

A-line styles

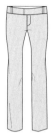

Straight-leg and trouser cuts

Bermuda or "city" shorts

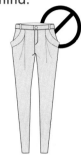

Tapered-leg styles, which exaggerate volume in the midsection

---

"Buy less, choose well."

—Vivienne Westwood

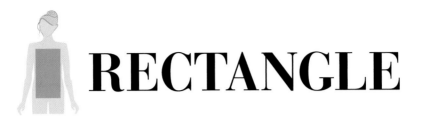# RECTANGLE

If your hips and shoulders are proportionate and your X intersects in the middle of your body, yet you appear to be straight all the way through, from top to bottom, you are typically considered to have a rectangle body type.

BODY BLOCKING

Dark Areas: Diminish with deeper colors, neutrals, solids, and vertical lines.

Light Areas: Draw attention to with bright colors, prints, texture, and horizontal lines.

As a rectangle, you can visually create your X by drawing the focus out to your shoulders and hips. Light, bright shades and high-contrast prints call attention, so wear these around your shoulders or hips to steal the spotlight, and let darker hues play a supporting role near your center. Seek out diagonal patterns, wavy prints, and designs that appear to flow with movement.

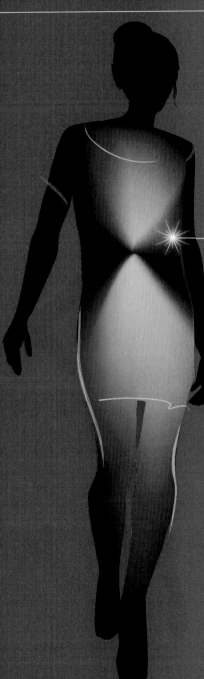

Ideal belt:
waist

BODY BLOCKING

IDEAL GOAL:
CREATE
CURVES

DRESSES

Carve Out Curves: Look for dresses that create shape and the illusion of a more defined waistline.

Look For:

Leave Behind:

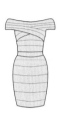 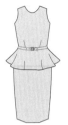 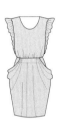 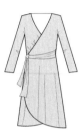 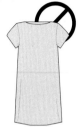

Fitted shapes and curved elements	Peplum styles	Tapered tulip designs	Wrap dresses	Boxy shift dresses, which offer no shape

TOPS

It's a Cinch: Mold your midsection with corset-type designs and wider belts.

Look For:

Leave Behind:

    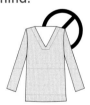

Ruched and gathered styles	Cowl necks and draped tops	Bustier and feminine fits	Off-the-shoulder and asymmetrical cuts	Square-cut tunics, which create a boxy effect

BOTTOMS

Define and Draw Attention: Look for pants, skirts, and shorts that add shape to your lower half.

Look For:

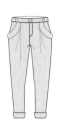

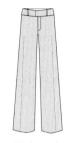

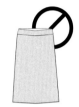

Bubble hems and tiered designs

Trumpet and flared styles

Pleated and tapered pants

Relaxed, wide-leg cuts

Square-cut skirts, which are shapeless

> "Clothes make the man.
> Naked people have little or
> no influence on society."
>
> —Mark Twain

FYI FOR ALL BODY TYPES

The long and short of it, for all of us, is that we need to master before we manipulate. Collecting guidelines

TIPS FOR PETITE FRAMES AND FULLER FIGURES

ELONGATE, STRETCH, AND LENGTHEN

- Vertical lines, seams, or detailing
- Monochromatic or low-contrast color combos
- Up-and-down prints and patterns
- Sleeves rolled or pushed up
- Empire-waist tops and dresses
- Shorter hemlines
- Pant creases, which lengthen
- Long necklaces, scarves
- Shoe colors that blend with skin, hosiery, or pants
- Shorter hairstyles, which highlight your neckline

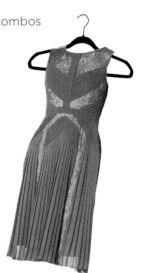

about your body type will help you understand your X factor, so you can then customize your individual needs. Regardless of your body type, whether you are short or tall, slight or full-figured, or somewhere in between, the following information will help you further balance your body.

TIPS FOR THOSE WHO ARE SLENDER AND/OR TALL

CREATE CURVES, MINIMIZE HEIGHT

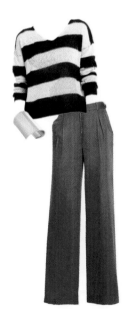

- Horizontal lines, seams, or patterns
- Separates and contrasting colors
- Larger-scale prints, which help fill out your frame
- Belted dresses to add a break
- Tiers, ruffles, and decorative hems
- Below-the-knee hems
- High-waisted bottoms
- Cuffed or cropped pants
- Narrow garments paired with wide garments, which creates curves
- Bold accessories, which favor taller frames

HIGH VERSUS
LOW CONTRAST

HIGH CONTRAST SEPARATES . . .
LOW CONTRAST STREAMLINES

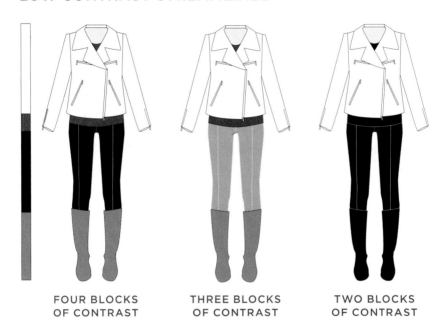

**FOUR BLOCKS
OF CONTRAST**

**THREE BLOCKS
OF CONTRAST**

**TWO BLOCKS
OF CONTRAST**

- Be creative with color and contrast. Use both to play with proportion and balance your body type.

- Grouping similar colors and tones together can visually blend on the body, while more variety can break things up.

- Points of low contrast will recede and fade, while high-contrast points will advance or draw attention.

ARM YOURSELF WITH INFORMATION

FLATTER SLENDER ARMS

Higher-cut armholes for hourglass, triangle, and diamond body types

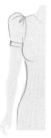 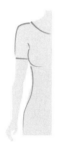

PUFF SLEEVE   STRAIGHT-CUT SLEEVE

FLATTER FULLER ARMS

Lower-cut armholes for inverted triangle and rectangle body types

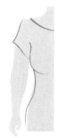 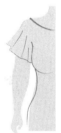

DIAGONAL-CUT SLEEVE   FLUTTER SLEEVE

UNIVERSALLY FLATTERING

FLATTER NARROW HIPS

Style tip: Don't dismiss chic and flattering longer lengths.

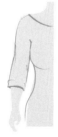 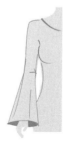

THREE-QUARTER-LENGTH SLEEVE   FLARE SLEEVE

UNIQUE TORSO TIPS

IF YOUR TORSO IS SHORT

- Leave tops untucked
- Cinch or belt lower around the hips
- Create balance with low-rise bottoms
- Choose A-line, empire, and wrap dresses
- Opt for three-quarter tops over leggings
- Accent with low-contrast, thin belts
- Elongate with low-contrast colors

IF YOUR TORSO IS LONG

- Tuck in tops
- Draw the eye higher with scrunched or cuffed sleeves
- Cinch or belt above the natural waistline
- Choose empire-waist tops and dresses
- Create balance with high-waisted bottoms
- Use bold or wide belts

Find your most flattering . . .

FOOTWEAR

Over-the-knee items: aim for them to reach the thinnest part of the thigh

Knee-high boots: opt for breathing room between the bottom of the knee and the top of the boot

Calf-high boots: boots that are dipped or angled at the top are elongating

Ankle straps & booties: inverted triangles and rectangles wear these well

Flats: consider toe shape

HEM

Thigh area: especially flattering for rectangles, inverted triangles, diamonds, petites, and stubbier legs

Just above to just below the knee: a universally flattering range for all body types

Mid-calf or "midi": will make all legs look thicker, for better or worse

Ankle-length hems: will make all body types appear shorter

Maxi length: below the ankle is flattering for all body types

TOE SHAPES

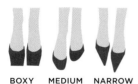

BOXY   MEDIUM   NARROW

Just like the X factor helps you balance your body with clothes, you can also bring your feet into the mix.

- Rectangles, triangles, and diamonds can slip into narrow, pointed, or sleek shoes, while avoiding square, overly round, or heavy toes, which can draw the eye down and cause a boxy effect.

- Hourglasses and inverted triangles can pull off heavier or rounder toes, as they can help visually balance a fuller bust or broad shoulders.

GIRLFRIEND SUPPORT

MINIMIZE A BUSTLINE WITH . . .

- A supportive bra
- V-, square, and cowl necks
- Solid tops and jackets in neutral or deep colors
- Vertical or diagonal stripes or details
- Wrap styles and tailored tops with darts
- Three-quarter sleeves, which flatter the most
- Jackets that button under the bustline
- Jackets and cardigans with deep shawl collars

MAXIMIZE A BUSTLINE WITH . . .

- A flattering bra
- Bright and light tops
- Horizontal stripes and prints
- Ruffled or pleated blouses
- Details at the bust (bows, ruching, etc.)
- Boat, crew, and high necklines
- Asymmetrical and bandeau tops (with support)
- Delicate jewelry

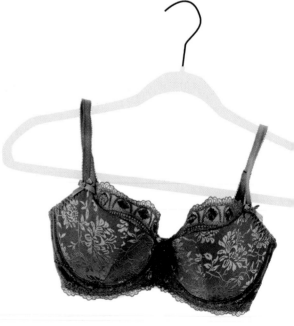

PREGNANCY

FLATTER YOUR FIGURE WITH . . .

- Cropped jackets and cardigans
- A-line and empire waists
- Flowing or fitted, *not* loose or baggy
- Layers and low-contrast colors, which elongate
- Wedge heels, boots, and fun flats

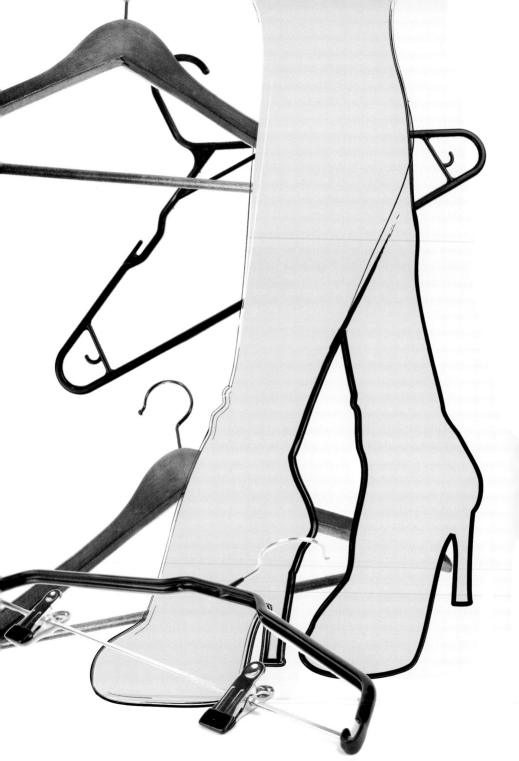

STEP EIGHT

PERFORM A CLOSET CLEANSE

The title of this step may not grab your attention the way it should, so imagine it's actually called "Where to Find Free Clothes Edited Perfectly for Your Personality in Your Best Colors and Most Flattering Silhouettes."

If you are like most of my friends, you've probably been meaning to tackle your closet for months. You may not realize it, but the benefits far outweigh the time investment. So why is cleaning out the closet something we tend to put off? Whether you admit it or not, it's usually because doing so forces you to address everything from body issues to buyer's remorse and make some tough decisions. You don't want to be reminded of how much money you spent on items you've never worn. Plus, you're reluctant to risk getting rid of something you may need in the future. You may also assign important memories to your clothing, and the idea of purging seems difficult. Whatever your prior excuses, you now have a better understanding of your best colors and the most flattering cuts for your body type, as well as a greater awareness of your identity and how to speak it with style. So you are more prepared than ever to review your current wardrobe from an informed perspective. As organizing expert Peter Walsh describes, "Memory clutter holds you in the past. I-might-need-it clutter holds you in the future. They both rob you of the present." *Now* is the time to employ everything you've mastered thus far and create your own personal dream store to shop in every day.

Consider the closet examples below. When looking at the closet on the left, does it make you feel anxious, overwhelmed, confused? What about the one on the right? Does it evoke words like "calm," "responsible," or "decisive"?

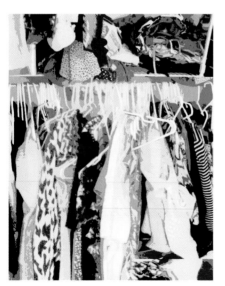 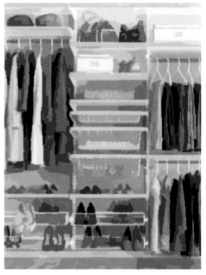

How do these two pictures make you feel?

Your closet can reveal so much. Never mind what someone else may think, should he or she be granted a peek behind the doors. How is your closet affecting *you* on a daily basis? Would you rather start your day feeling anxious and overwhelmed or calm and organized? A lot of people use their closets as a place to throw clothes in order to get them out of the way. (Better than the floor, right?) But where you keep your clothing greatly affects how you approach dressing for your day. Just because your closet is out of sight doesn't mean it should be out of mind. Much like a tidy, well-stocked kitchen makes you more likely to cook, having an organized, easy-to-navigate closet space makes getting ready more fun.

I'm not saying you need to hire an interior decorator or a professional organizer, or build a new wing off your bedroom just for your clothes. No matter what type of closet you have, you can make the most of your space. Simply spending some time organizing will contribute to the feeling of having a "new" wardrobe and help reignite and re-energize the way you look at your clothes. By cleaning out your closet, you cut through any excess clutter and create a calm, organized space, which will give you the freedom to be more creative with your clothes and, ultimately, your style.

IF YOU CAN'T SEE IT, YOU WON'T WEAR IT

How many times have you either felt or said aloud "I have nothing to wear"? Chances are you were standing at the time in front of an overstuffed closet or set of drawers that barely shut. But the thought of sifting and searching for something to wear is a workout in itself.

Throughout any closet cleanse, it's important to keep this in mind: if you can't see it, you won't wear it. You have to leave enough room in your closet for your clothes to breathe. I typically know it's time to reorganize when I find myself forcibly shoving hangers in between others, occasionally breaking one or two in the process, or when I notice that a dress or shirt doesn't even need a hanger to keep it from falling to the floor. If you know what I'm talking about, you have too many pieces for your space and likely aren't seeing what's available to you. I know it can be tough to let go, but believe me, downsizing will make a difference. Don't fall victim to the black hole of an overstuffed closet. It's time to get in there and make some room in your wardrobe.

How to Detach and Decide

Cleaning out your closet isn't something anyone necessarily wants to do, which makes it that much harder to set aside the time. And while I would like you to pull everything—and I mean *everything*—out of your closet piece by piece, I promise you my strategy is simple and will make the process as painless as possible. The idea is you're going to *quickly* decide if each item is a yes, no, or maybe, and toss it into a corresponding pile. Keep an efficient pace—try not to take more than a few seconds to choose—and allow your initial knee-jerk reaction to inform you as to which pile to place each item in. Overall, go with your gut. Yeses and nos should be instantaneous. And if you are having trouble determining what to do with a particular piece, consider it a maybe. If it helps, you can repeat this rhythm in your head: *one, two, three, four, if I'm not sure, maybe.* Here are some quick tips to help you decide your yeses and nos.

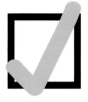

Yes: Those articles you wear most often. Your go-to, I've-just-worn favorites and special-occasion pieces. The things you know fit perfectly and you definitely don't want to be without. Keep in mind your style-speak objectives and fight the urge to put everything in your yes pile. Doing so will only make the closet cleanse less effective.

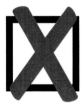

No: The items you haven't worn in over a year or didn't wear at all the last time they were in season. If it doesn't fit, or you forgot about a stain you meant to remove, or you can't remember the last time you wore it, odds are you won't miss it.

Once you've gone through everything, the yes pile goes right back into your closet, while the no pile can be bagged up and ready for donation. This strategy helps you divide and conquer, because you instantly eliminate two of the three piles, leaving behind a manageable maybe pile.

You have now created a situation where you are in control. You've made a sizable dent and felt the instant gratification that comes with accomplishment. And a big bonus: you are able to see the space you still have to work with, which will help guide you as you sort through what remains. If you're still energized, continue tackling the maybe pile, or if you need a break (or have a hot date), put the pile aside for later, when you can come back with a fresh perspective. That's why this approach is easy.

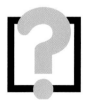

Manageable Maybe: This pile is the hardest to attack, since it's comprised of all the things you didn't immediately want to let go of but are on the fence about whether you really need.

Fit Comes First!

One rule: Before any maybe can become a yes, it must be tried on. I start with this rule because we're all only human. It stands to reason that you may have been ten to twenty pounds lighter ten to twenty years ago. If that's the case, and you're considering holding an item for "inspiration" to get back in shape or lose weight, I can empathize with how much work goes into this endeavor. So I would rather your inspiration be that you reward yourself with a new pair of jeans or dress instead. The exception to this is if it's a special investment item or one with sentimental value, but be realistic (e.g., you last wore it a decade ago or before you got pregnant). If the sentimental item isn't being worn or is unrealistic, you can always label a bag up in the attic or storage space CLOTHES ELIZ HAS AN EMOTIONAL ATTACHMENT TO, **like my illustrator Elizabeth has.**

I recommend going through this group an hour at a time every week. This way the process won't feel as intimidating or time consuming. If you find yourself plucking a piece from the maybe pile to wear within the first few days, consider it a yes. If you can go a month or more without missing something, move on and make room for something better. When considering each item, be sure to ask yourself "How often will I wear this?" and "Is it worth the space it will take up in my closet or dresser?" Also consider the comfort factor. What kind of first impression would you make in the piece? If it doesn't fit right or you recall being uncomfortable the last time you wore it, it will show in your body language and it's time to toss.

Turnaround Tip

If you hang all your maybes back in your closet with the hanger hooks facing out, when you wear one, replace it facing in. Then you'll know what you actually wear!

Though cleaning out your closet may feel at first like you're eliminating options, by editing yourself you're actually ensuring that every day will be a great fashion day. It stands to reason that if you keep only the best, you'll always look your best. Personally, I prefer

STYLE SESSION

Flatter Yourself!

Everyone has, at the very least, one item that needs a tweak. While you may not be able to buy all your clothes custom-made, you can make your clothing custom. Grab from your maybe pile that item you love and haven't tossed even though it needs a new zipper, or the too-long, loose, boxy, etc. pieces worth saving. Fit is everything, so find an affordable tailor who can make the needed alterations. Even if something is too tight, short, ripped, or stained, you'll be amazed at what a talented tailor can fix. Rather than investing more time and energy eternally searching for the perfect blazer, pair of jeans, etc., make something you like perfect for you. Basic alterations, often costing less than twenty dollars, can make a major impact.

to have fewer amazing pieces that I love than a wardrobe jammed full of impulse buys. So in the future, don't forget to keep room in your wardrobe. For every new purchase, consider letting something else go to maintain balance—the magic word. Extra closet space will encourage you to coordinate and combine different items, make updates, and even pack more efficiently. So remember, out with the old and in with the new, so you're always able to see what you own and make clear, informed decisions when getting dressed.

REWORK YOUR WARDROBE

Once you've sorted through your clothing, downsizing enough to actually see everything you have, it's time to finally bring order to your closet. Have you ever noticed how department stores and clothing boutiques work hard to visually welcome you? They neatly organize and cleverly display their merchandise in order to present their items in the best possible way. After all, the goal is for shoppers to be attracted to the products enough to purchase them. When shopping is an enjoyable experience, it's something you'll want to repeat. Well, you can take a few notes from your favorite stores and give your closet a boutique feel by merchandising what you own the way stores do. By incorporating a few of their simple tips and tricks, you'll stay in control of your clothes and not slide back into any old habits.

Group by Garments: Make sure you keep similar items together (i.e., dresses, skirts, shirts, sweaters, and pants should all be separated by type). If you want to take it a step further, you can subdivide each garment type by hem or sleeve length. When you put something back into your closet, take the extra few seconds to make sure it's in the proper place.

Color-Coordinate: Next, go through each garment group and organize by color. Not only is it more aesthetically appealing, it will also help you immediately find what you're looking for.

Stack to Save Space: Sweaters and jeans can take up a lot of room in your closet, so stack these items in a way that makes sense. Separate sweaters by cable knits, cardigans, turtlenecks, etc., and make sure to place the bulkiest on the bottom. For jeans, you want to be able to identify which pair you're looking at without pulling it out of the pile. You can mark your shelves with tape according to style (bootcut, flare, skinny, etc.) and then create a color-graduated stack. Remember to keep all stacks around eight to ten inches high to prevent toppling.

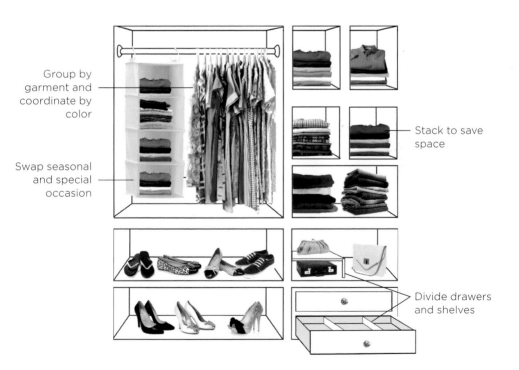

Group by garment and coordinate by color

Swap seasonal and special occasion

Stack to save space

Divide drawers and shelves

Divide Your Drawers and Shelves: Your intimates drawer is often an afterthought, where most people just toss bras, panties, and hosiery to keep them out of sight. Invest in a few drawer dividers to keep these items separated and prevent your foundations from forming a tangled mess. This will also keep a dreaded bra hook from tearing holes in any of your delicates.

Swap Seasonal and Special Occasion: Stores display only what's in season and so should you. Items like ski jackets and bathing suits are often kept in closets year-round. But unless you live in an area with a static climate, this takes up space for pieces that won't be worn for months out of the year. The same can be true with formalwear or special-occasion pieces. Pick up a few hanging shelves that can fasten to a closet rod and keep these seasonal or situational items in separate storage (not in your closet) when they aren't in use. Then, when their season rolls around, you can easily swap one hanging shelf for another (e.g., swap your bathing suits and sarongs shelf for the one housing your hats and scarves).

DRESS YOUR DRESSING AREA

Now that you've revised, why not refresh? While these may seem like finishing touches, consider making some small updates to your closet space throughout the cleansing process.

- **Light and Bright:** Closets by nature are often looked at as dark cubbies, so make sure yours is well lit and inviting. Apply a fresh coat of bright white paint to the inside (stay away from drab, darker colors), and add extra lighting to make your clothing stand out. If you don't have an overhead light in your closet, try applying a few battery-powered, stick-on LED lights to illuminate your space.

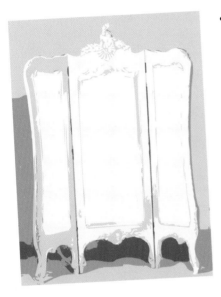

- **Mirrors:** A quality mirror (not warped, bent, or tinted) near your closet, which allows you to see yourself full length, will help you efficiently style looks. I'm continually baffled by hotel rooms (and a few friends) that rely only on vanity mirrors above the bathroom sink. Lean a mirror against a nearby wall or affix one to the inside of a closet door. If possible, create a 360-degree view by angling mirrors next to each other.

- **Helpful Hangers:** Invest in uniform hangers; keeping them all the same will help you see your inventory without being distracted.

- **Sitting Space:** If you have the room, create a sitting area in or outside your closet. As in stores, it's all about comfort and convenience when trying on clothes.

- **Mood Music:** Keep your stereo or iPod speakers near your closet area. Music can lift your spirits and get you in the groove before a busy day or a fun night out.

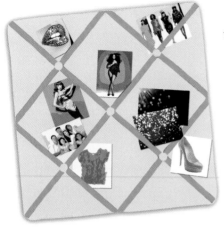

Don't be afraid to add personal touches to your closet. After all, it's an extension of you filled with your essence. Whether you pin up inspirational pictures or mount a memo board where you can keep your most-wanted list or reminders of what you wore to a special occasion, the goal is to turn your closet into a place you'll want to spend more time.

ASSEMBLE YOUR ACCESSORIES

When it comes to accessories, creative storage is key. By containing and consolidating, you make it possible to see, store, and sort through all your belongings. You can pick up helpful storage systems at most home goods stores, or you can repurpose items you already own to create custom solutions.

Make It Easy

Having easy access to all your accessories is half the battle to staying organized. Tangled jewelry and hard-to-see handbags are less likely to be worn than those items within arm's reach. And it's easier than you may think to take full advantage of everything you own.

Jewelry: There's nothing wrong with an old-school jewelry box, but if you've outgrown yours or are in need of a better way to see what you have, one of my personal favorite finds is the hanging

Preserve and Protect Your Pieces

While sorting through your stuff, you'll notice that some of your items are in need of a little TLC. Over time, colors fade, sweaters pill, and shoes and handbags lose their shape. If you feel like you could be taking better care of your clothes, here are some helpful items to keep handy and tips to keep in mind.

Items to have on hand

- Wrinkle-release spray or a garment steamer to fight folds without an iron
- Boot shapers and handbag forms to maintain shapes (or use empty wine bottles for boots and cardboard or newspaper for bags)
- A dehumidifier or desiccant packs to keep your closet dry in humid environments
- Color-protecting detergent for bright clothes and a gentle version for delicates
- Stain sticks and/or spot-removal kits
- Sweater bricks to remove fuzz

Tips to keep in mind

- Remove plastic wrapping and dry-cleaning bags, as they can cause yellowing and weaken a fabric's fibers.
- Avoid hanging knits, wovens, and delicate items on hangers, as they can become misshapen and risk snags and holes.
- Never, ever put away clothing that is still damp from a dryer, etc., as it will mold, stain, smell, and possibly bleed or change color.

pocket organizer. These organizers are beloved by TV and film stylists, who use them on set; you can hang one inside your closet door and the clear pouches will help you easily find earrings, brooches, watches, and more.

Handbags: There are hundreds of ways to store handbags. I've learned from experience that stacking purses on top of one another can ruin their shape, and shoving them into bins can be just as bad. Invest in a simple shelf divider to keep your bags safe and within your sight. You could also use a household item you already own, like a dish divider or stacking rack from the kitchen. Both are great tools for separating handbags on a shelf. This way, when you pull one out, your entire collection of carryalls won't come tumbling down.

Belts and Extras: While it's commonplace for people to use shoe organizers to store their soles, they can also come in handy to hold belts or to hide your special-occasion extras under a bed. The individual compartments keep everything separated and easy to spot.

Be Resourceful

While most simple storage items are relatively inexpensive, I'm a big fan of the motto "waste not, want not" and feel strongly that you don't necessarily have to buy anything new in order to better organize your closet. By being resourceful, you can repurpose things from around your house and turn them into excellent storage solutions. I can all but guarantee you have a few of the following items lying around just waiting to be transformed.

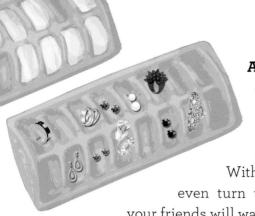

An Extra Ice Cube Tray or Plastic Egg Container: Both of these can be used to sort rings, small earrings, etc., and can be stacked in a drawer. With a little spray paint, you can even turn them into creative containers your friends will want to try for themselves.

Common Candlestick Holders: These decorative accents can double as a pretty way to display bangles and bracelets, getting them out in the open where you are more likely to add one to your outfit on your way out the door. (You could also use paper towel holders.)

Slat Rack or Ladder: For items like scarves and ties, you can get creative with a slat rack, ladder, or trellis. Whether it's no longer used in your garden or a leftover from your children's old bunk beds, you can weave your long layers through the holes or rungs and lean it on a wall or behind a door for a crafty way to keep these accents in order.

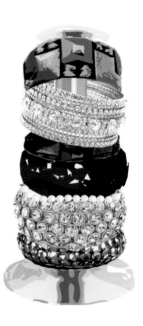

DIY and Display

Another clever storage trick is to turn your accessories into art. This way, instead of trying to find space to hide your tiny treasures, you can showcase your jewelry with a crafty case or stand. After all,

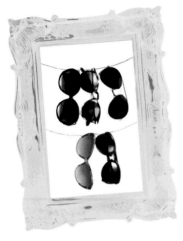

whether on you or on your dresser, these pretty pieces are meant to be seen.

Frame Your Frames: Picture frames are a great way to hang sunglasses or even earrings. Just remove the glass, and stretch rope, twine, lace, or wire mesh (found at a craft store) across the frame's edges. You can hang glasses along the rope, twine, or open-patterned lace, or hook earrings into the mesh.

Store Your Silver: Cutlery boxes aren't just for silverware. They can easily be transformed to display your necklaces. Simply line the box with anything from placemats to wrapping or contact pa-

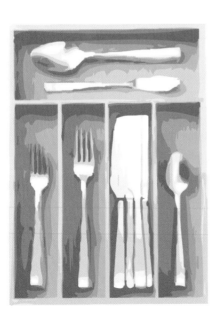

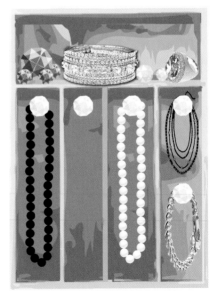

per, even wallpaper scraps, then tack small nails or little knobs inside and you're all set. An alternative idea for those who want a readymade solution: a plethora of inexpensive jewelry stands are available at discount department stores and can make beautiful, decorative statements.

Performing a closet cleanse is as much an emotional exercise as it is a physical one. Maintaining a sense of outer order contributes to inner calm, and you are worthy of the time it takes to create a beautifully organized closet space. You will feel lighter, inspired, creative, and in control. As we've discussed, the choices you make when you first open up your closet for the day, or week, will send messages to everyone you encounter and affect many of the opportunities that come your way. This butterfly effect begins in your closet, so give yourself an advantage and transform your wardrobe space into your own personal sanctuary. Because getting dressed should be an experience you look forward to.

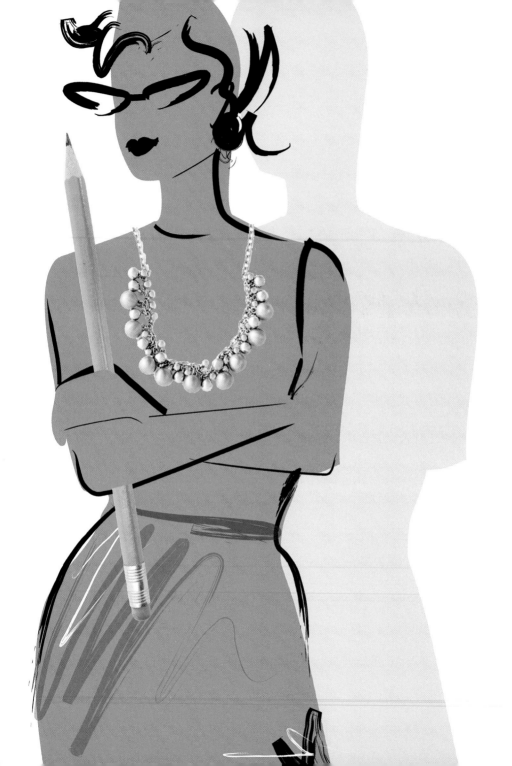

MAKE A MOST-WANTED LIST

In life and with style, you sometimes have to break things down in order to better build them back up. Your closet cleanse did this. By performing a physical (and emotional) purge, you are now in the perfect position to become your own best stylist. I'm excited for you to survey everything you've kept with a fresh, insightful perspective and use these pieces to make powerful, personal statements that best communicate who you really are. Yet in order to do this effectively, you'll need to gauge not only what you currently own, but also what you may still need. Together, we'll make a most-wanted list of items, which will help you develop a signature wardrobe. Open your laptop, smartphone, or tablet, or pick up an old-fashioned pad of paper (my personal favorite) and jot down notes, thoughts, and a running tally of your wants.

Open your laptop, smartphone, or tablet, or pick up an old-fashioned pad of paper (my personal favorite) and jot down notes, thoughts, and a running tally of your wants.

In the first half of this book, I asked you to think about your reflection, the first impressions you make, and what you wanted others to know about you, all to see yourself as a brand. Keeping you the brand in mind, try to come up with a quick style ID: a mental objective or tagline you feel best captures who you are and what you want to say. It could be a few words à la "practical, polished, and playful" or a mission statement like "I'd like to dress for the job I want, not the job I have." Your style ID should be easy to recall and will help you keep your closet and your most-wanted list on track.

Your Style ID

Jot down your style objective:

_____

_____

_____

_____

_____

Whatever inspires you, write it down and display it somewhere in your closet where you'll be able to see it. Now, with this ID as your reminder, we're going to walk through three exercises aimed at seeing your clothes differently. When you're through, you'll have identified only those most-wanted items that meaningfully contribute to your wardrobe.

FIRST, TAKE INVENTORY

Evaluate

At this point, I'd like you to evaluate your current wardrobe, keeping in mind your style ID, color compass, and X factor. While everything in your closet may be a yes, it's important to take a step back and really see what you're working with. Looking at the big picture, can you call out any ruts your style has fallen into or areas that need improvement? Maybe you have an abundance of jeans and it might be time to dress things up a bit. Perhaps you have only one or two skirts suitable for work. If you have twenty-five pairs of yoga pants, it could be a sign that you should finally take up yoga. Or you may discover most of your stock is the same color, explaining why you occasionally feel bored by your options. (Don't be surprised if you even find you want to let go of a few original yeses.) Take note of any obvious "wants" and add them to your list. Here are some helpful questions to spot any themes:

- Is there a common color category or shade (black, browns, neutrals)?

- Do you own mostly solids, prints, or a combination? Are the prints similar (say, all florals)?

Create an "I Wore, Why, Buy" Log

An easy way to find out what you actually wear from your wardrobe, and how often, is to create a simple log. You'll need three columns: I Wore, Why?, and Buy? Over the course of thirty days list your outfits or key items. You don't have to be obsessive about it, and it doesn't have to be every day, but whenever you think about it—at work while drinking your coffee, before you get ready for bed, or while watching TV—jot down the following information.

I Wore The main items you wore—whichever dress, skirt, shirt, pants, shoes, and any accessories. If you're logging the past week, note how often you repeated an item in that week.

Why? Your reason for choosing each one. It may be due to a special occasion, because you like the way it fits or flatters, because it's the only one you have, or because it pairs really well with other pieces—just a few words to help you pick up on your patterns. You might notice that a certain item is worn numerous times because it's filling a gap, or you wear a specific dress or skirt more than others.

Buy? What you need to buy, based on what you wear and your reasoning. If you wear a go-to basic (e.g., a specific T-shirt) multiple times in a month, you might want to consider buying another to have when that one's dirty, or picking up some additional colors. If you notice you often don a certain dress, think about investing in another of the same cut. Or use this column to remind yourself of something needed to complete a look or wear it a new way (e.g., a brown belt to make those pants feel more casual or new pumps with more polish to elevate this skirt for work). This will help reinforce your style-speak needs.

Keep this log somewhere convenient—a closet shelf, nightstand, purse, or desk drawer—so it's easy to update. After a month you'll have a thoughtful and specific record of items to add to your most-wanted list. You'll also have an idea of what you may not need to keep and what you may want to invest more or less money in. (Step 10's "Consider Cost per Wear" section will help inform you about these items as well.)

I wore...	Why?	Buy?	
My long black stretch tank top 3x this week	I love the fit, and it's the only one I have that's long.	The same one in other colors?	>>> FIT FAVORITE
My bright coral linen scarf	It's soft, keeps me warm at work & adds a fun twist to everything.	Quirky, bright-colored cardigans? Lime? Teal?	>>> PERSONALITY PREFERENCE
My blue jeans	They let me wear all my delicate blouses without feeling too "girly."	Menswear-inspired trousers?	>>> COST PER WEAR

Please Wear

If you're like me, there's a good chance you came across some beloved "I forgot I had that" or "Why haven't I worn this?" items when cleaning out your closet. For your forgotten favorites, you can create a special PLEASE WEAR column or separate list to remind you. This could also alert you to potential reasons that you haven't worn the item (e.g., you don't have the right shoes or a top or bottom to match).

- Do you own more of one garment type than any other (all pants and only two dresses)?

- Is there a dominant item (many ivory blouses or ten pairs of black pants)?

- Are your pieces mostly pull-on and stretchy or tailored and crisp?

While the closet cleanse cleared the clutter, this assessment reveals your dressing habits, shopping routines, and more. You may have been wanting to go out with girlfriends lately but now realize you haven't followed through because you don't have what you would want to wear (darn those yoga pants). Be open and honest with yourself, because this evaluation is personal and based on your unique lifestyle. Only you can identify and decide what your specific wardrobe needs are, so call attention to anything you notice is missing or underrepresented in your current clothing collection. Add these items to your most-wanted list.

Catalogue

You've now had the opportunity to step back and get a bird's-eye view of your belongings and to determine any general themes or ruts, and have hopefully added a few key items to your most-wanted list. Next, it's time to get down to the nitty-gritty. Before we go any further, let me stop right here and stress that you'll have to do this only once, so look at it as a short investment of time now for a tremendous return later.

Okay, with that said, I'd like you to consider creating a "look" book: a visual directory of your wardrobe made up of snapshots of all your pieces of clothing. A more literal way of taking inventory, a look book is intended to help you discover specific items you may need in order to complete full looks and really round out your stock. Take a photo of each item in your closet, whether on a hanger, laid on your bed, or laid out on a sheet on the floor. It can be helpful to snap pictures in a mirror of yourself wearing the pieces to remind you of the fit or of complete outfits you like. You could even find images online, either of the exact item or something similar (e.g., search for "black wrap dress"), to get the gist of what you have.

Once you've captured your collection, the rest will just be maintenance. Add a photo only when you buy something new or want to be reminded of an outfit. If you have a smartphone, I recommend taking the images with your phone and uploading them directly to your computer, where they can be stored in a separate file, but you can easily take them with a point-and-shoot camera as well. Much more effective than simply looking through your closet, where you are more likely to miss something, this physical record can be grouped into categories based on clothing type, occasion, or whatever makes the most sense for you.

In a perfect world, you'd be enthusiastically engaging in the weekly fittings I suggested back in step 5, but I realize it's extremely likely that one morning you'll find yourself in bed wondering what to wear. If your look book lives in a file on your desktop at work, that's not going to help you decide, is it? This is why I suggest that you print it out (*gasp*) to really kick-start your good habits. Having a hard copy you can keep in a nightstand or dresser drawer will help make your clothing decisions (and packing plans) exponentially easier. You can even jot down notes on the back of each image with a particular style-speak adjective, or list other items you like to pair with that piece, creating outfit ideas that will guide you when dressing for a specific occasion.

If you do this, I guarantee you will thank me the next time you have to go to a wedding or an important meeting, when you'll be able to flip through your look book of options, pre-approved to accurately reflect you and your style speak. I understand if you're hesitant, especially if you're in your teenage years and your closet could completely change by the next season. But if you're older and into a groove at this point in your life, creating a look book will give you a snapshot of items you'll likely own for years to come. Adding another picture only after a new purchase will let you visually watch your wardrobe evolve as you do.

> "It's a new era in fashion—there are no rules. It's all about the individual and personal style."
>
> —Alexander McQueen

SECOND, SHOP YOUR OWN CLOSET

Once you've identified any general themes or holes in your wardrobe and created a go-to look book of what you have, you're more than ready to go "shopping" in your own closet and get creative with combinations. Creating outfits will inspire you to add more useful wants to your list. You've organized your closet to look like a store, so now you can shop it like a store! Just like you would approach building a new outfit from the shelves and racks at your favorite boutique, go into your closet and get inventive.

Find Inspiration: Revisit your style file from step 3, and look at any images you collected. From pictures of friends and celebrities to Pinterest profiles, magazine ads, and more, notice if there are any looks or variations of looks that you can re-create using what you own. I mentioned a few favorite movies (*Annie Hall*) that have informed my style choices over the years. Rewatch yours and take style notes. If you have a specific fashion icon, it's not impossible to steal her style. Celebrities don't have their own secret stores, and even though they do have big bank accounts, oftentimes they or their stylists just know how to combine basics, colors, and shapes in unique ways. If you're drawn to an ad, a store display, or an amazing ensemble someone else is wearing, take note of details, such as layering, lengths, color combinations, whether the pants are cuffed or the sleeves are rolled. Then reconstruct your own version. If you feel like your version doesn't look exactly the same, make sure you've adjusted for your X factor, keeping in mind that you may need to alter an element or two. If you find inspiration in a home décor picture, try mixing pieces that have similar textures, colors, or prints. Remember to keep your phone or camera handy to add to your look book and show the different possibilities you've created.

Blend Your Basics: Many women are guilty of mentally separating their professional and personal styles. Don't divide your closet into work and nonwork pieces. It's possible to find balance and blend your look with basic key pieces. For example, the blazer is a work staple that can easily become a weekend favorite by pairing it with more casual items on your days off. A polished jacket takes on a whole new look when you fold the cuffs, scrunch up the sleeves, or wear it with a loose-fitting unisex T-shirt and relaxed jeans. Don't separate your work wear from the rest of your closet; incorporate it.

Pairing Seasonal Items: Make your wardrobe work year-round by mixing and matching warm- and cool-weather pieces. You can wear summer dresses into fall by pairing them with cardigans or layering cozy sweaters over similar soft, flowy frocks. Heavy accessories, like leather boots and winter tights, will complement lightweight pieces by adding contrast. And if you pick the deepest colors from a spring or summer floral pattern, then pair it with chocolate brown, charcoal, or black, rather than ivory or beige, you will bring out a warm fall feel.

See Yourself Through Someone Else's Eyes

Ask a friend, your mom, your sister, or even the guy in your life for some feedback. You can try on new ideas of your own or ask them to play stylist and pull together a few looks for you. (I often ask this of those closest to me. It's more interactive, plus it's fun to watch how a loved one would dress you!) Also, if you're unsure about what an item might be saying, when considering your style ID and overall style speak, it's helpful to have another person share the first few words that come to mind when he or she looks at it.

THIRD, ADD THE EXTRAS

While you've made thoughtful additions to your most-wanted list thus far, there could still be an item or two you have yet to think of. So just in case you're asking "How do I know what I'm missing, if I don't know what I'm looking for?" I encourage you to start thinking like a stylist. Consult the following lists for suggestions of items you may still be in need of.

✓ Clothing

☐ **The Little Bold Dress** Whether it's black or your favorite color, invest in a flattering fit you can reinvent as needed.

☐ **An Effortless Dress** A zip-and-go option that looks and feels easy, can be dressed up or down, and works for both day and night.

☐ **A Soft Blouse** A fluid top that will instantly add elegance or ease to anything you pair it with.

☐ **A Tailored Button-Down** Whether it's worn crisp or casual, this versatile classic adds polish.

☐ **Basic Tops** Alone or layered, simple T-shirts and long-sleeve tops are essential to any wardrobe.

☐ **Layering Tanks** Great for low-cut or sheer tops. Consider buying seamless stretch tanks in black, a shade that matches your skin tone, and possibly a few of your favorite colors. Plus, longer tanks will offer extra coverage over leggings.

☐ **Dress Pants** From slim straight cuts to trouser styles, a flattering pair of basic black pants will offer a solid canvas for all types of tops.

☐ **A Flatter-Your-Figure Skirt** A timeless silhouette in black or another sophisticated solid will provide you with a base for pairing both trendy and classic tops.

☐ **Casual Pants** Black leggings, yoga, or soft cargo pants look comfy chic rather than lazy compared to alternatives such as sweatpants or pajama-style bottoms.

☐ **Light and Dark Denim** If you own only two pairs of jeans, opt for both a light and a dark hue for maximum versatility. Consider gray as your next neutral option.

☐ **Classic Shorts** Invest in a neutral-colored pair of a flattering length.

☐ **A Cardi-Wrap** An effortlessly chic, go-anywhere, wear-with-anything layer.

☐ **A Chic, Structured Blazer** Black is a safe bet, but navy, gray, or camel can also pull anything together, from jeans and a T-shirt to a soft dress.

☐ **A Trench Coat** Not just for rainy days, this is a timeless style that can add polish to casual looks, yet it's chic enough for dresses.

✓ Shoes

☐ **Nude or Flesh-Colored Shoes** Heels, sandals, or flats in your skin tone.

☐ **Pretty Pumps** Whether you invest in black or a fun color, just be sure to have a pair of heels that make you happy.

☐ **Fun Flats** Whether they add a pop of color or are made of an on-trend print, fabric, or material, flats are an easy way to make a comfy and stylish statement.

☐ **Riding Boots** Not too casual and not too dressy; just right for so many outfits.

✓ Accessories

☐ **Two Classic Handbags, One Light and One Dark** Your dark could be black, brown, or burgundy while your light could be blush, camel, or white; whatever works for your style speak.

☐ **Smaller Purses** From clutches to mini cross-body bags, keep an on-the-go assortment. Consider basic black, anything-goes metallic, or even a vibrant print, which can be surprisingly versatile.

☐ **A Statement Scarf** Whether it's a solid pop of color, your favorite animal print, or a studded show-stopper, a scarf can be worn and styled in countless ways.

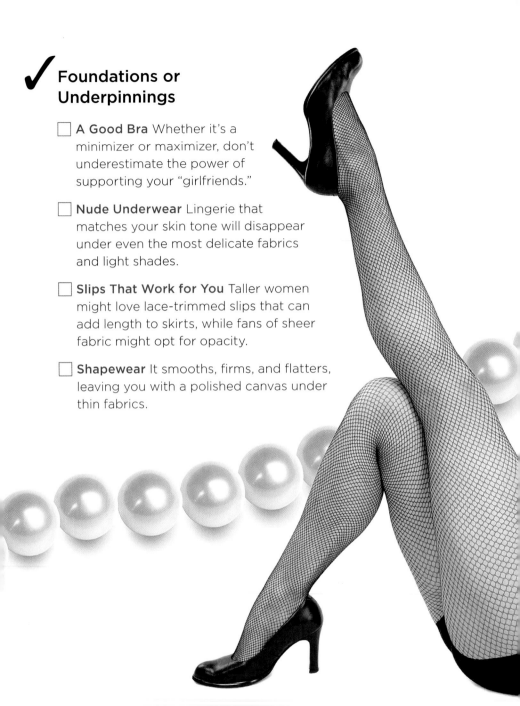

✓ Foundations or Underpinnings

- ☐ **A Good Bra** Whether it's a minimizer or maximizer, don't underestimate the power of supporting your "girlfriends."

- ☐ **Nude Underwear** Lingerie that matches your skin tone will disappear under even the most delicate fabrics and light shades.

- ☐ **Slips That Work for You** Taller women might love lace-trimmed slips that can add length to skirts, while fans of sheer fabric might opt for opacity.

- ☐ **Shapewear** It smooths, firms, and flatters, leaving you with a polished canvas under thin fabrics.

✓ Go-To Styling Kit

A good styling kit can save you from any number of fashion catastrophes. I recommend making sure you add any essentials you don't already own to your most-wanted list. Trust me, it's better to be safe than sorry, so stock up on these style savers for when you need them most.

- [ ] **Safety Pins** To close gaps, hide holes, and tighten waistbands.
- [ ] **Small Pair of Scissors** For loose threads and uncomfortable tags.
- [ ] **Double-Sided Tape or Fashion Tape** To prevent straps from slipping, close gaping blouses, or fix a hanging hem.
- [ ] **Silicon Nipple Covers** Reusable, to control pesky, perky moments.
- [ ] **Deodorant Sponge** To remove any accidental marks left on darker clothes (never use a damp cloth!).
- [ ] **Lint Roller** Especially important for anyone with pets.
- [ ] **Sweater Stone or Fabric Shaver** To remove pilling on overly worn fabrics.
- [ ] **Antistatic Spray or Fabric Softener Sheets** To prevent your clothes from clinging.
- [ ] **Mini Sewing Kit** For any loose buttons, tiny tears, etc.
- [ ] **Travel Steamer** To keep your clothes wrinkle-free on the go, heats up quickly in a pinch.
- [ ] **Shoe Inserts** Make new shoes more comfortable or fix the fit of heels that are stretched out or too large.

OPPOSITES ATTRACT

Sometimes an outfit just doesn't feel right. You keep trying every possible top you own to make a bottom you want to wear work. It's often the case that you need to go in the opposite direction. For any pieces that you're not sure how to wear, consider the following styling suggestions for inspiration on what you may need to make it work for you.

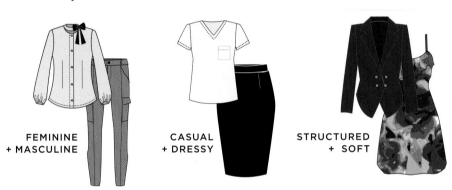

FEMININE
+ MASCULINE

CASUAL
+ DRESSY

STRUCTURED
+ SOFT

STYLING AND STYLE SPEAK

Stylists are great at thinking outside the box and figuring out how to make one basic piece say different things based on how it's styled. Take another look at some of your favorite pieces and, considering your style ID and style-speak adjectives, see if you can creatively envision what you might need in order to style that piece so it says what you want it to. Anything you don't already own can be added to your list.

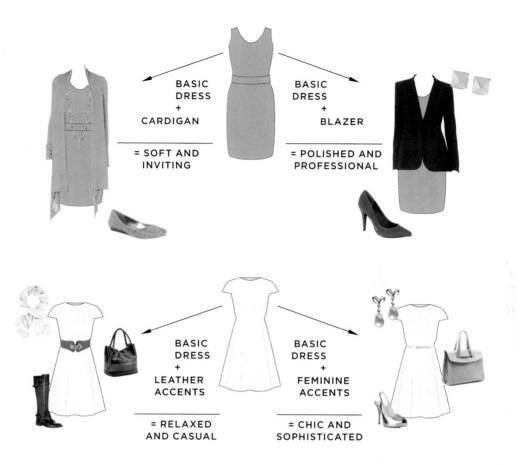

BASIC
DRESS
+
CARDIGAN
———
= SOFT AND
INVITING

BASIC
DRESS
+
BLAZER
———
= POLISHED AND
PROFESSIONAL

BASIC
DRESS
+
LEATHER
ACCENTS
———
= RELAXED
AND CASUAL

BASIC
DRESS
+
FEMININE
ACCENTS
———
= CHIC AND
SOPHISTICATED

While I hope you now have a better sense of items you want, and need, that doesn't mean you have to run out tomorrow and buy everything. It's called a most-wanted list because it will give you purpose and priority. Rank your list in order of importance, and be sure to really use it. Instead of aimlessly shopping, you now have direction. You no longer have just something to wear but what you *want* to wear.

Now, finally, let's go shopping!

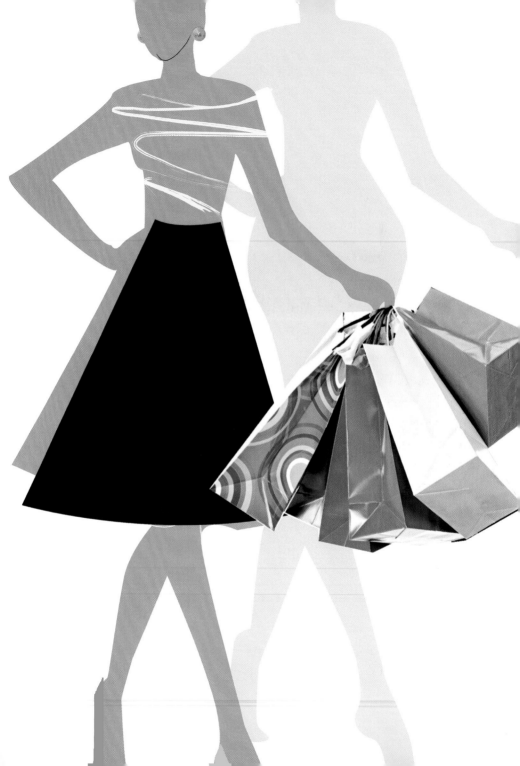

LET'S GO SHOPPING!

While "retail therapy" is a phrase used to describe the temporary high that comes from purchasing something new, the truth is this feeling often fades after the first time you wear whatever new thing you've bought. But when you consciously approach shopping with purpose, you're likely to feel this same rush every time you go into your closet, because all your items will have intention. So without further ado, the time has come to confidently add value to your well-edited wardrobe. Grab your most-wanted list and get ready to put into play your style-speak goals, color compass, and unique X factor, because you're heading out into the field!

SHOP SMART

While it's commonly assumed all women love shopping, a recent report by WGSN (Worth Global Style Network) found that 28 percent of women actually hate it. While I am part of the enjoy-shopping crowd, it's not terribly difficult to understand why some women don't feel this way. It could be due to the expenditure of money, the amount of time it can take, the crowds, or any number of other factors, but shopping can and should be a positive experience. The end result is powerful, ultimately enhancing and refreshing your style as well as helping you better express yourself and attract what you desire in return. Whether you view shopping as a chore or an art form, consider it a necessary skill. Now let me help you be the best shopper you can be.

Here are a few things to keep in mind no matter where you shop.

Less Is More: Buy fewer but better. Be extremely selective and carefully consider what you buy, so you eliminate the endless questioning in front of your closet or mirror at home. If you're unsure, leave it behind. Rest assured, something you can't stop thinking about will lure you back. Most important, by making the decision up front, you will have a wardrobe full of items that you are completely confident about, align with your goals and go-to adjectives, and you will love wearing.

Don't Be Suckered by Sales: Never buy something on sale you wouldn't pay full price for. It's not a bargain if it isn't great.

Buy Multiples: As we mentioned in step 9, "Make a Most-Wanted List," if you find the perfect piece and notice you wear it often, buy more than one. Be it a pair of jeans, a shift dress, or a T-shirt, you can stick with the exact same version or pick it up in other colors.

Invest in Solids: When buying a pricey investment piece, stick with solids over trendy prints or patterns. Unless it's a classic pat-

Consider Cost per Wear

When setting your budget, make sure you factor in cost per wear. If you were going to wear the same outfit every day for the next year, how much would you spend on it? Well, you wear your hair 365 days a year, so how much are you willing to spend on a great cut and color? Do you invest in a classic coat you'll wear all winter or opt for an expensive dress or necklace you'll wear to only one or two big events? How much time are you willing to spend on your body or on finding the perfect make-up and skincare for your specific skin type? You wear items like shoes and handbags repeatedly, whereas you may wear that sequin skirt only once. Everyone is different and your Achilles' heel might be a current trend, like neon accessories or harem pants, and that's fine. Just pay attention to the fact that these things, while attention grabbing, are less likely to be permanently woven into your wardrobe. So if you're trying to stick to a budget, also be mindful of trying trends from the most affordable places.

tern (like stripes or dots) or the item is a special signature piece that you love and can't imagine not splurging on, it's easier to wear solid colors past their original season.

Stick to Your Budget: I recommended in step 5 that you create a style budget for your seasonal wants and needs. You can even include a reserve amount for unexpected finds you come across. All in all, have a plan and stick to it. If it helps, carry cash only.

That way once you've spent it, you know it's time to head home. Remember *you are worth it*. Your image is a priority, so be strategic about how you spend.

Avoid Emotional Shopping: While a trip to the mall might sometimes sound like just what the doctor ordered, avoid shopping when you're depressed or down in the dumps. Never shop to fill a void. Only buy pieces because you love them. Emotional shopping is as unsatisfying as emotional eating, so resist the urge to impulse-buy and binge-shop.

INSIDER TIPS

I feel like everyone has that one friend who always finds the greatest clothes, gets the best deals, and figures out just where to shop and when to shop there. She knows the mall better than the back of her hand and has all the trendiest online retailers bookmarked. Well, this friend likely isn't part of any secret club or elite, underground shopping fraternity; she just knows the insider tips and uses them to her advantage. You can easily be this person by learning the best ways to approach both in-store and online shopping.

In-Store

One reason window-shopping is such a treasured pastime is because the physical act of going to a store allows you to see, touch, and try on almost anything your heart desires. Under no obligation to buy, in-store shopping offers you the opportunity to take a

Departments Defined

The different sections of a department store can create confusion among even the most seasoned shoppers. The simple explanation is that the sections each carry clothing cut to fit different body types. So what's the difference between Juniors and Misses, Women's and Pluses?

Juniors: These clothes are created for younger bodies that have fewer curves and less definition between the bust, waist, and hips. Aimed at teens and those in their early twenties, this section typically carries casual, trendy items. Sizes run in odd numbers from 1 to 13.

Misses: For women with more developed curves, these items are cut to fit the common eight- to ten-inch difference between a woman's waist and hips. With options ranging from sportswear to formal to business, sizes usually run in even numbers from 0 to 20.

Petites: While it's a common misconception that this department is reserved for women who are particularly small and slight, it's actually all about height. The Petites section typically carries clothes for those five feet four and shorter, of most shapes and proportions. Sizes run similar to Misses, from 0 to 20, but with shorter inseams and hemlines.

Pluses: This section is aimed at full-figured women with larger hips and busts (who usually need larger than a D-cup). Sizes typically run from 1X to 5X.

Women's: Not as common today as it once was, Women's is for the more mature women (usually sixty years and over) and cut to be comfortable and allow more mobility. Today, women of all ages still want to be fashionable, so this category is slowly falling out of favor. Size numbers are accompanied by a *W*.

break from the real world and browse the many beautiful displays. And while shopping can definitely be a great social experience, my number one personal rule when it comes to shopping at brick-and-mortar retailers is to shop with friends but buy alone. Sure, from friends you'll often gain valuable second opinions and helpful suggestions on items and outfits, but even with the best of intentions, your friends don't always know what's right for you. Opt to put things on hold and take time to think before you buy. Flying solo gives you the opportunity to stick to a plan, take your time, or even stay in the dressing room half the day, if that's what it takes, all without the pressure of worrying about someone else's timetable.

> **Shop with friends but buy alone.**

In addition to my number one rule, there are plenty of other helpful insights to take note of before you head out on your next shopping trip:

- Stay in control. Shop the store; don't let the store shop you. You are in charge of what you purchase, so don't be afraid to leave empty-handed if you don't find what you're looking for. Never allow friends or salespeople to talk you into anything you aren't sure of.

- Bring to the store bags of your own items to help you finish a look or match a hard-to-wear piece. And be sure to keep your most-wanted list handy.

- Don't go if you're tired or hungry.

- Shop early. Stores are neater and more organized in the morning, and the clerks are more alert and attentive.

Tips for Trying On

Although the dressing room is a haven of private space, it can turn into a personal hell. If you have experienced a fitting-room failure because of harsh lighting, a bad hair day, or the genius idea to try something on after a buffet lunch, here is some additional food for thought:

- Dress to undress. Wear something you can quickly zip on and off and shoes you can slip in and out of. And put your best face forward (with a little makeup) to set yourself up for success.

- Wear skin-toned lingerie, as it will fade away rather than distract, and appropriate shapewear if you're looking for items you intend to use support with.

- Keep the jewelry to a minimum so you don't accidentally leave it behind when changing or snag it on delicate pieces.

- Have a pair of heels or a belt stashed in your bag to give you a better idea of a complete look.

- Evaluate your choices not only in your dressing room but outside in the shared mirror, and move around to ensure you can comfortably walk and sit in whatever you are considering.

- Not to sound like Mom, but it's a good idea to test zippers, etc., and look for marks or stains in the mirror.

- Whenever you find yourself in a fitting room feeling not so great, that's the time to reach into your wallet or peek at your phone for the uplifting stickie note you wrote yourself back in step 1. Smile, give yourself a break, and focus on what you *do* like about that reflection looking back at you, instead of what you don't.

- Ask about restocking days. You'll find new items and a better selection of sizes, and you'll be the first to see new discounts.

- Stay on top of sales. Many weekend promotions start on Thursdays, so visit the store's website or Facebook page prior to your trip. Ask about VIP or frequent-shopper cards, and check if there is a smartphone app or instant coupon available.

Fun Facts

- Studies show that consumers tend to veer to the right when first entering a store. Therefore, retailers stock their most expensive items on this side.

- Ever wonder why the perfume department is always front and center on the ground floor of a department store? Scent heightens our saliva glands, which makes us much less disciplined shoppers.

- In a pinch, you can get a good idea of whether a skirt or pair of pants will fit by wrapping the buttoned or zipped garment around your neck. If you still have a thumb's worth of wiggle room, it will likely fit your waist.

- For major excursions, use valet parking, if possible and affordable, or look into having items delivered or shipped. If available, rent a locker or ask a store clerk or service desk to hold your items while you finish.

Online

While there are plenty of people who still prefer the overall in-store shopping experience, there is a lot to be said for shopping from the comfort of your own computer, tablet, or even smartphone. Instead of getting dressed, gassing up the car, and taking time out of your day to travel to the store, the Internet brings the stores to you. With the world at your fingertips, the process may be faster and more convenient. Online shopping allows you to browse an infinite range of products and purchase items from all around the globe. Also, you typically have a more defined idea of what you're looking for when you head to the web, making impulse splurges less of a concern. But before you hit the cyber waves, there are plenty of tips to consider.

- **Comparison-Shop:** Look for search-engine sites that allow you to shop multiple stores in one place, enabling you to seek out specific items, desired details, price points, etc. A few of my faves are ShopStyle.com, HomeofFashion.co.uk, SnapFashion.co.uk, WeareverYouAre.com, and good old-fashioned Google.com/shopping.

- **Ship:** It's smart and convenient. Have items sent straight to your home, so you can try them on in front of your mirror and with your existing wardrobe and accessories. Just be sure to look into

Beware of . . .

Hidden Fees: Some sites don't mention high shipping fees until the second before you click BUY. Pay attention to your total cost to ensure you aren't overpaying. If possible, have the site ship to the nearest physical store location to avoid shipping fees altogether.

Sloppy Sizing: Whether you're shopping from a boutique website or that of a larger chain, be aware of sizing discrepancies. Not all stores share the same size charts, and since you won't be trying anything on, be sure to consult the one specific to the site.

Poor Pictures: Some companies still don't invest in high-resolution images for their products and, sadly, computer screens can make it difficult to really see the quality or true color of an item. If you don't get an accurate idea from the photo, proceed with caution.

Payments and Passwords: Be sure to use a separate password for shopping sites, and I strongly suggest designating one credit or debit card (preferably one with a controlled limit) for your online purchases so you're not sharing sensitive information. Plus, from the common AVOID HITTING THE PAYMENT BUTTON TWICE message to confusion over whether your purchase went through, pay attention when checking out, and keep all contact information along with a screen capture of the transaction, if possible.

any shipping or restocking fees. Most reputable stores want your business and try to make returns free and easy, so consider buying extra sizes or colors to ensure fit.

- **Get Codes and Coupons:** Scan the Internet for e-coupons and discount codes. You may be able to find special offers for free shipping or a percentage off. Just make sure the information you're getting is reputable. Never give your personal information to an unknown third-party site.

- **Read the Reviews:** A helpful shopping tip unique to the Internet is the ability to read reviews about the items you want to purchase. Rarely will a helpful stranger magically appear before you in line at a boutique to tell you that the dress you're about to buy won't withstand the washing machine or that the shoes you just tried on will stretch out after one wear. So read the customer reviews, if available, and take into account what people are saying before you buy.

- **Shop Direct:** Companies that design brands sold at larger retailers, yet don't have their own brick-and-mortar stores, often have e-commerce stores on their websites where you can find exclusives and other options.

Shopping Alternatives

Last but not least, not all of your shopping must be done at the mall or online. There are many other budget-friendly and eco-conscious ways to expand your wardrobe.

Resale and Consignment: Everything old is eventually new again. There are amazing deals to be had and items to be found at vintage stores, thrift shops, and even flea markets. It might take a little more digging, but I've unearthed many gently used gems that I cherish. Not only do these items offer you a break from mass-produced pieces many others own, they can also help you save money and be eco-friendly by recycling. However, if you dread the bargain hunt, you'll find that many boutiques list their inventory online and have done much of the editing for you.

Swap Parties: We all have items we once loved but for whatever reason no longer wear, or items we thought we would love but don't wear, even though we keep convincing ourselves we *might*. Well, if you and all your friends have a few of these pieces (see step 8, "Perform a Closet Cleanse"), have a swap party! After all, they say one woman's lightly worn dress/shirt/skirt or accessory is another woman's treasure. Swap parties offer up an opportunity to get together with friends, score free fashions, and know that your beloved clothing is going to a good home. You could also go online to find community swap parties or websites that let you swap with women elsewhere.

Host Your Own Swap Party

It's fun and easy to host your own swap party. All you need are a few friends and a handful of clothing items you no longer wear. Follow the steps on the following page for great swapping.

1. Pick a day, time, and location and send out an invite (an e-mail, Facebook event, or snail-mail invitation, depending on your preference). Ask everyone to RSVP, so you have an idea of how many items will be available for swapping.

2. On the scheduled day, set out some snacks or ask friends to bring their favorites and make it a potluck. Whether it's a weekend brunch with coffee and bagels or an evening affair with champagne and cupcakes, a few light bites are always welcome.

3. Play some tunes to inspire: RuPaul's "Supermodel," Right Said Fred's "I'm Too Sexy," Roy Orbison's "Pretty Woman," Babyface's "Incredible," and so on.

4. As the women arrive, for every item they bring, give them a colored ticket or index card or Post-it note that corresponds to one of the below four categories, then place their items on the correct category pile or table.

   - Low for low-priced items
   - Mid for medium-priced items
   - High for high-priced items
   - Deal or No Deal for items they're willing to barter

5. Have each woman write her name on the tickets she's been given and toss them all into a bowl.

6. The host will pick out three names and those women get to "shop" the collections that match the color of their tickets or barter, trading up or down (e.g., two Lows for one Mid).

7. Repeat the process until all the items are gone and all deals are made.

Shop His Closet: Menswear-inspired pieces have been in vogue for years, so why not borrow a few items from a guy in your life? Your brother's, boyfriend's, husband's, or roommate's button-down, with the sleeves rolled, belted or left loose over leggings can give you an instant Annie Hall look. Or add a few masculine accents, like one of his belts (tied in a knot if too long), an oversize watch, a silk pocket square, or his cozy cardigan to reinvent your basics.

Earlier, in step 2, I questioned whether shopping was a woman's birthright. Frankly, it's everyone's birthright, but I hope you now understand that it's so much more than that. Shopping should not be considered a trivial pursuit but rather a search for the meaningful and substantive. If you respect shopping as an opportunity to thoughtfully select what will help you communicate to the world, you'll be rewarded with true style.

> Shopping should not be considered a trivial pursuit but rather a search for the meaningful and substantive.

MATCH THE MIRROR

There is only one you, and nothing is more worthwhile than understanding who you are and being able to share this knowledge with others. By guiding you through your unique style process and arming you with personalized information, I hope I have helped you now be able to align all the things about yourself that can't be seen with those that can. In doing so, you will continually put your best, most accurate self out into the world.

Think back to the style session in step 1 called "Who's That Girl?" when I asked you to take an honest look at yourself so you could identify your self-perception. Well, take another look in the mirror. My hope is that you now see what you *do* like—that you notice all the positive aspects of yourself represented in the specific style choices you've made echoing back to you in that reflection. From this point on, I want you to look in the mirror and love what you see. It's not an easy task, as you know, but it's 100 percent possible and my wish for you.

Most important, remember that the true power of style is self-expression. Achieving it is a journey, one that takes effort and commitment. But trust me, it's worth it. Whenever I have the opportunity to speak to those who embrace the significance of their personal image, I try to remind them that caring about the superficial (in the literal sense) isn't shallow or frivolous; it's simply good business, since some of the most consequential areas of your life may depend on it.

It's a lesson I'm constantly reminded of at the *TODAY* show, where I sometimes feel like the fluff segment of an esteemed program packed with a parade of pop-culture icons, Oscar-winning actors, respected journalists, and even dignitaries. One day I was having one of these existential moments in the makeup room, sandwiched between former president Jimmy Carter and journalist Matt Lauer. As Matt adjusted his dapper necktie and Jimmy Carter leaned forward to fix his hair in a well-lit mirror, I smiled, reminded that personal image isn't everything . . . but it's often the window to everything.

10 STEPS TO MATCHING THE OUTSIDE TO THE INSIDE

Awareness: Your Internal Makeover

1. SEE YOURSELF

Remember: *Work on manifesting a healthier image. Don't approach a mirror on a seek-and-destroy mission. Use the mirrors around you (your friends, your home, the way you carry yourself) to brilliantly reinforce and reflect your best qualities.*

2. ACT THE PART

Remember: *Body language is the only constant form of communication. Over 90 percent of communication is nonverbal, so be aware of what your body language, demeanor, and overall style are saying about you. Make sure your verbal and nonverbal messages are in sync. Pay attention to how people react to you when you first meet them and what they are reacting to. Use nonverbal communication to reinforce, not compete, with your personality, goals, and interests. Appearances matter.*

3. SPEAK UP

Remember: Your style is a layer of language you wear, communicating on your behalf and being perceived by others. Consider yourself a brand worthy of accurate promotion, and understand who you are and what you want to say. Use your style speak to pinpoint your message based on your goals and intentions.

4. KNOW YOUR WORTH

Remember: Make sure you are placing your value in constant, intrinsic qualities that can't be taken away. Accept yourself and know that you're worth the time, energy, and effort it takes to invest in yourself and your packaging. And share your gifts with others.

5. PUT A PLAN INTO PRACTICE

Remember: You are your own priority, and input equals output. So put effort into committing to your own style journey. Set a style budget, find time for fittings, and conjure up an ideal version of you as your goal.

Execution: Your External Makeover

6. LEARN YOUR COLORS

Remember: Understanding whether you are warm or cool and creating a custom color compass will help you use color to make your most flattering style statements.

7. BALANCE YOUR BODY

Remember: You only have one body, so learn how to dress it in ways that will highlight your best attributes. Knowing your unique X factor will assist you in choosing clothes that work best for your body type.

8. PERFORM A CLOSET CLEANSE

Remember: Keeping your closet clutter-free will eliminate extra style stress and make the everyday process of getting dressed easier and more enjoyable. Follow the tips suggested to ensure that you stay in control of your closet.

9. MAKE A MOST-WANTED LIST

Remember: Your clothing speaks for you, so make sure you identify the items you wear most often and why. By keeping a thoughtful most-wanted list, you will guarantee that any new clothing choices reinforce who you are.

10. LET'S GO SHOPPING!

Remember: Shopping is not a trivial pursuit, but rather a search for the meaningful and substantive. Understanding the best times to shop, common retailer tricks, how to tackle dressing rooms, and more will help you get the most from your shopping experience.

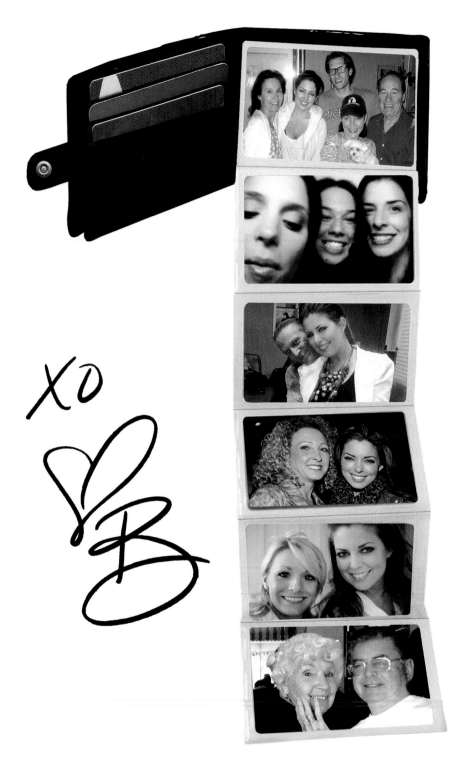

XO

B

Acknowledgments

They say it takes a village to raise a child, and for the past five years, this book has been my baby. It would not be what it is without the help, love, and support of everyone in my personal "village." My gratitude to the following people goes beyond these words.

First, thank you to my family. To my mom, Fatima, whose unconditional love has guided me throughout my life and has given me the courage to pursue my passion. To my father, Robert, who instilled my drive; my sister Eileen, who has laughed and cried with me; and Alexi, who cared for me as his own and blurred the conventional role of stepfather. Also to my remarkable grandmothers, Alice and Arminda, who I'm lucky to still have with me. To Lester, Vivian, and Sara, for all of their TLC along the way. And especially to Michael—a man of profound character and unrelenting patience who accepts all of the crazy elements of my life, and has made room for them in his.

Thanks to my best friend and "gubby," Lash Fary, one of the most creative and stylish people I know, who devoted countless hours and was the first to help me put my thoughts on the page. To my second mom, Lynn Harless, who is unapologetically honest and has been an inspiration to me. A constant source of support from the moment I met her, she continues to be my number one lifeline today. To hair expert extraordinaire, Rita Hazan, for all of the help (and highlights) she's given me over the years and for always being my saving grace in those last-minute moments of panic. Thank you to Stacy Ferguson, aka Fergie, who heard so much of this book in its rawest form back in the day in her Mustang . . . butterfly girl, we have spread our wings.

Maggie Murray, you are my unsung hero who could . . . (finish my sentences), and I owe rent to you for sharing a brain. This book would still be on Post-it notes, scrap paper, and in some document I can't find or open if it wasn't for your wit, patience, and unique ability to understand all sides that elevated this manuscript beyond my expectations.

To Mike Plotkin, someone who is a little bit psychic, never wrong, and so much more than my lawyer. His encouragement and wisdom have opened my eyes and more doors than I could have ever dreamed of. Michael Mesnick, affectionately known as "the guy who keeps the lights on," thank you—lol, it's hard to write in the dark! And then there's Richard Spencer, who accepted my first column (via fax) handwritten on a paper towel and *still* offered me an opportunity that changed my life—something I'll never forget.

I feel incredibly lucky to have such an amazing and talented support system at Creative Artists Agency: Stephanie Pacuillo, Peter Hess, Katie Maloney, Ashley Davis, Amy Yavor, Peter Jacobs, and especially the wonder woman who is Lauren Hale—super-smart meets supermodel meets super-person to have in your corner, both personally and professionally. I adore you. I also owe a special debt of gratitude to Ted Harbert, Benny Medina, Alan Berger, and Andy Stabile, who first helped me navigate the industry and introduced me to my phenomenal book agent, Gary Morris. I can say with confidence that there are few in this business as patient and open-minded as Gary, and who really understand the meaning behind the phrase "thinking outside the box."

To the coolest editor a girl could ever ask for, Jeanette Perez. From our initial Skype meeting and my instant girl-crush, and throughout the entire book process, my gratitude and respect for you know no bounds. From the bottom of my heart, thank you for "getting it." And of course, to all the other geniuses at HarperOne who brought *The Power of Style* to life: Jacqueline Berkman, editorial assistant; Mark Tauber, publisher; Claudia Boutote, associate publisher; Darcy Cohan, director of publicity; and Suzanne Quist, manager, production editorial.

I wouldn't be where I am today without my *TODAY* show family. Words cannot express how much I've learned from my spirit guides Kathie Lee Gifford and Hoda Kotb, who have both on- and offscreen rooted for, cheered, advised, encouraged, and embraced me. And thanks to the entire cast of rock stars, including but not limited to Megan Kopf, Brittany Schreiber, Elena Nachmanoff, Tammy Filler, Jaclyn Levin, Matt, Meredith, Al, Ann, Natalie, Savannah, Sara Haines, Rachel Alves DeLima, Cecilia Wang, Jim Bell, Don Nash, Debbie Kosofsky, Adam Miller, Marc Victor, Amy Rosenblum, Dee Dee Thomas, Rina Raphael, Jen Brown, Gerry, Ed, April, Laura, Mary, Donna, and the crew with the biggest hearts in the business.

Last but not least, to my girls, "Team BT"... where do I start? I am humbled by your ingenuity, skills, and never-ending support, and I'm privileged to play the role of wizard in our Oz. Stefani (Tsakos)

Vlasopoulos, we've long surpassed being coworkers or friends and should sign the paperwork, as we are officially sisters—you've worked tirelessly to help me shine and without hesitation have enlisted family and friends to serve (thank you, Chris, Irene, Andria, and Roula). Elizabeth Romaner, you are not only the intern who became indispensable, but you are now a valued part of our team and a young woman filled with limitless talent, as evidenced by your artwork on these pages. I still wonder if you eat or sleep, because you have been there for me 24/7—thank you (ditto from Chica). To the small army of smart, hardworking, and energetic girls who have volunteered their time and enthusiasm as interns over the years, thank you. You have all in unique ways reminded me why I love what I do. And to Andrea Abraham DeVos, who has been willing to try/wear anything, fly away with me on a moment's notice, and partake in companion calories—I'm so excited about what's to come!

Credits

Unless otherwise noted, photographs are courtesy of the author.